Frontiers in Periodontology - New Directions and Emerging Therapies

Edited by Elna Chalisserry

Published in London, United Kingdom

Frontiers in Periodontology - New Directions and Emerging Therapies
http://dx.doi.org/10.5772/10.5772/intechopen.1000465
Edited by Elna Chalisserry

Contributors
Aikaterini-Elisavet Doufexi, Faten Kafa, Federica Di Gregorio, Fowziya M. Ali, Gianluca Monaca, Giovanni Assenza, Giovanni Barbagallo, Gloria Alì, Kolovou Stolina, Konstantinos Papadimitriou, Lourdes Alfaro-Ochoa, Luis M. Maita Castañeda, Luis V. Maita Véliz, María M. Castañeda Mosto, Neophytou Chariklia, Pitu Wulandari, Rebeca Sánchez-Martos, Santiago Arias-Herrera, Vanina Porto

First published in London, United Kingdom, 2024 by IntechOpen
IntechOpen is the global imprint of INTECHOPEN LIMITED, registered in England and Wales, registration number: 11086078, 167-169 Great Portland Street, London, W1W 5PF, United Kingdom

British Library Cataloguing-in-Publication Data
A catalogue record for this book is available from the British Library

Additional hard and PDF copies can be obtained from orders@intechopen.com

Frontiers in Periodontology - New Directions and Emerging Therapies
Edited by Elna Chalisserry
p. cm.

This title is part of the Dentistry Book Series, Volume 19
Topic: Oral Health
Series Editor: Sergio Alexandre Gehrke
Topic Editor: Sandra Marinho and Esra Guzeldemir-Akcakanat

Print ISBN 978-0-85466-935-6
Online ISBN 978-0-85466-934-9
eBook (PDF) ISBN 978-0-85466-936-3
ISSN 2631-6218

For EU product safety concerns:
IN TECH d.o.o., Prolaz Marije Krucifikse Kozulić 3, 51000 Rijeka, Croatia,
info@intechopen.com or visit our website at intechopen.com.

IntechOpen Book Series
Dentistry
Volume 19

Aims and Scope of the Series

This book series will offer a comprehensive overview of recent research trends as well as clinical applications within different specialties of dentistry. Topics will include overviews of the health of the oral cavity, from prevention and care to different treatments for the rehabilitation of problems that may affect the organs and/or tissues present. The different areas of dentistry will be explored, with the aim of disseminating knowledge and providing readers with new tools for the comprehensive treatment of their patients with greater safety and with current techniques. Ongoing issues, recent advances, and future diagnostic approaches and therapeutic strategies will also be discussed. This series of books will focus on various aspects of the properties and results obtained by the various treatments available, whether preventive or curative.

Meet the Series Editor

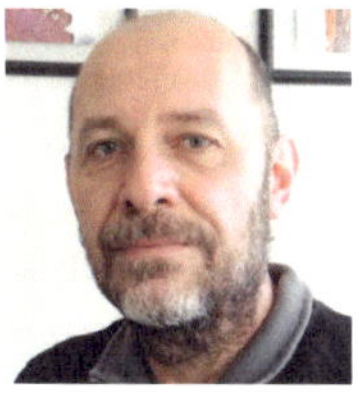

Dr. Sergio Alexandre Gehrke is a doctorate holder in two fields. The first is a Ph.D. in Cellular and Molecular Biology from the Pontificia Catholic University, Porto Alegre, Brazil, in 2010 and the other is an International Ph.D. in Bioengineering from the Universidad Miguel Hernandez, Elche/Alicante, Spain, obtained in 2020. In 2018, he completed a postdoctoral fellowship in Materials Engineering in the NUCLEMAT of the Pontificia Catholic University, Porto Alegre, Brazil. He is currently the Director of the Postgraduate Program in Implantology of the Bioface/UCAM/PgO (Montevideo, Uruguay), Director of the Cathedra of Biotechnology of the Catholic University of Murcia (Murcia, Spain), an Extraordinary Full Professor of the Catholic University of Murcia (Murcia, Spain) as well as the Director of the private center of research Biotecnos – Technology and Science (Montevideo, Uruguay). Applied biomaterials, cellular and molecular biology, and dental implants are among his research interests. He has published several original papers in renowned journals. In addition, he is also a Collaborating Professor in several Postgraduate programs at different universities all over the world.

Meet the Volume Editor

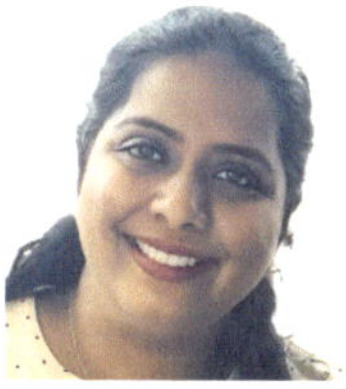

Elna Chalisserry is currently an adjunct assistant professor at Pushpagiri Research Centre, India. She obtained her bachelor's degree in Dentistry from India and subsequently earned a master's degree in Oral Pathology from Queen Mary University of London. Dr. Chalisserry was awarded her Ph.D. from Pukyong National University, Busan, Korea. She has held roles as a researcher and assistant professor at King Saud University in Riyadh and Jazan University in Saudi Arabia, respectively. With more than 12 years of experience in research, Dr. Chalisserry has made significant contributions to the field of dentistry, particularly in developing biofunctional biomaterials for bone regeneration and exploring the therapeutic potential of stem cells. Her work has extended to the field of periodontology, where she has focused on the use of novel biomaterials and regenerative techniques to enhance periodontal healing and bone regeneration. Dr. Chalisserry has published extensively in peer-reviewed journals and contributed chapters to books, sharing her expertise on these topics. She has also presented her research at various international conferences and workshops, particularly highlighting her innovative approaches to bone regeneration in different animal models.

Contents

Preface

This book provides a comprehensive overview of the latest advancements in periodontal and peri-implant disease management, aiming to bridge gaps in current knowledge and enhance clinical and research practices. The collection addresses key themes such as the integration of innovative therapeutic strategies, the potential of regenerative medicine, and the use of advanced technologies in periodontal care. It explores the adjuvant effects of probiotics in modulating the oral microbiome, the role of epigenetics and stem cells in promoting periodontal regeneration, and the transformative impact of emerging technologies like three-dimensional printing and laser therapies. These discussions emphasize a shift towards minimally invasive and patient-friendly approaches, highlighting new methods for diagnosis, treatment, and prevention that prioritize safety and efficacy.

The volume is particularly timely and relevant in today's context, as the field of periodontology continues to evolve with rapid scientific advancements and technological innovations. It addresses the growing demand for evidence-based, non-surgical treatment options that align with contemporary clinical practices and patient expectations. Furthermore, it provides insights into novel non-invasive evaluation techniques, contributing to more accurate and safe assessments of periodontal conditions. By bringing together these diverse topics, this volume offers a rich resource for clinicians, researchers, and students, equipping them with the knowledge needed to navigate the complexities of modern periodontal therapy.

The necessity of this volume lies in its ability to consolidate recent findings and emerging concepts that have the potential to reshape periodontal practice. As the understanding of periodontal diseases expands, there is a critical need for resources that not only present the latest research but also translate these findings into practical, applicable knowledge. This volume aims to fulfill that need, serving as an indispensable guide for those seeking to stay at the forefront of periodontal research and clinical care.

I extend my heartfelt thanks to my mentor, Prof. Anil Sukumaran, for his constant support and invaluable guidance, which have been instrumental in shaping this work. I am also deeply grateful to the contributing authors for their significant input and to the publishing team for their dedicated efforts in bringing this volume to fruition. This work stands as a testament to the collective expertise and commitment of all those involved, providing a vital contribution to the field of periodontology.

Elna Paul Chalisserry
Pushpagiri Institute of Medical Sciences and Research Centre,
Thiruvalla, India

Section 1

Foundations and New Perspectives in Periodontal Health

Chapter 1

New Approaches in Etiology, Diagnosis, and Treatment of Periodontal Disease

Neophytou Chariklia, Kolovou Stolina,
Konstantinos Papadimitriou and Aikaterini-Elisavet Doufexi

Abstract

Dentistry is under continuous progress. Especially periodontal research and new therapeutic approaches have been developed in the last decades. The mechanism of periodontal disease development, diagnosis, classification system, and treatment protocol are disputed. At the same time, genetics with single-nucleotide polymorphisms (SNPs) signify the role of predisposition in periodontal disease. The relationship between periodontitis and systemic health is considered as an uncontested reality, and comorbidities with other diseases have been proved. Some recent advances and future perspectives in treatment field are immunomodulation, prebiotics, and vaccines, while biomaterials, like emdogain, and minimal invasive surgery are evolved frequently in periodontal treatment. This chapter presents and analyzes the total progress and changes in every aspect of periodontology from the past to now and the future.

Keywords: periodontology, periodontal disease, classification, genetics, minimal invasive surgery, biomaterials, immunomodulation, prebiotics, vaccines

1. Introduction

Periodontology is the field of dentistry that concerns the supporting tissues of teeth. In the last years, periodontology has been evolved, and numerous advances are in progress. For example, in the past decades, periodontitis, the infectious disease of gingiva, is considered as a degenerative disease, while now it is proven that it is caused by bacteria. Moreover, the classification system of periodontitis has been modified, based on recent knowledge about progression of the disease, predisposing factors, and state of periodontal destruction.

We conducted a search on the electronic database PubMed, Cochrane, and Scopus up to December 2023. We used as keywords the terms we referred previously.

2. New classification and its application

The previous classification system for periodontal diseases, established in 1999, gave rise to uncertainties and divisions within the dental community. Coupled with the exponential growth of knowledge in recent years, there arose a necessity for a revised classification system that would be more user-friendly, reflective of the latest insights into the etiology and progression of periodontal diseases, and adaptable to evolving clinical practices. To address these needs, a collaborative effort between the American Academy of Periodontology (AAP) and the European Federation of Periodontology (EFP) convened the World Workshop on the Classification of Periodontal and Peri-implant Diseases and Conditions in Chicago from November 9 to 11, 2017, with preliminary discussions commencing in early 2015 [1].

This organizing committee oversaw the creation of 19 review papers and four consensus reports, covering various facets of periodontology and implant dentistry. The task assigned to the authors was twofold: to update the 1999 classification of periodontal diseases and conditions and to formulate a corresponding framework for peri-implant diseases and conditions. Additionally, reviewers and workgroups were tasked with defining relevant case scenarios and establishing diagnostic criteria to aid clinicians in applying the new classification effectively. The outcomes and recommendations of the workshop were reached through consensus agreement among the participants.

Herein, we present a brief overview of the modifications introduced compared to the 1999 classification.

The workshop addressed unresolved issues from the previous classification by delineating between the presence of gingival inflammation at individual sites and the definition of a case of gingivitis. Consensus was reached that bleeding on probing should serve as the primary indicator for setting thresholds for diagnosing gingivitis. Furthermore, the workshop provided clear definitions for periodontal health and gingival inflammation in cases of reduced periodontium following successful periodontal treatment. Specific criteria were established to distinguish between cases of gingival health and inflammation post-treatment, based on bleeding on probing and residual sulcus/pocket depth. This differentiation underscores the importance of comprehensive maintenance and monitoring for patients successfully treated for periodontitis. It was acknowledged that while a patient with gingivitis can revert to a state of health, a patient with periodontitis remains so for life, necessitating lifelong supportive care to prevent disease recurrence. Additionally, the workshop reorganized the classification of non-plaque-induced gingival diseases and conditions based on primary etiology.

Concerning periodontitis, the workshop recognized three identifiable forms: necrotizing periodontitis, periodontitis as a manifestation of systemic disease and the conditions previously categorized as "chronic" or "aggressive" periodontitis, now consolidated under the single category of "periodontitis." This consolidation was accompanied by the introduction of a multidimensional staging and grading system for periodontitis. Staging primarily considers disease severity at presentation and the complexity of disease management, while grading provides supplementary information regarding the biological features of the disease, including historical disease progression, treatment prognosis, and its potential impact on overall health. Staging comprises four categories (stages 1 through 4), determined by various clinical parameters such as clinical attachment loss, bone loss, probing depth, presence of bony defects, tooth mobility, tooth loss attributed to periodontitis, number of teeth loss, and complication of a case. Grading encompasses three levels (grades A, B, and C) and incorporates factors such as the patient's general health status, smoking habits or metabolic control in diabetes, as far as disease progression, allowing clinicians to tailor treatment plans accordingly. For a comprehensive understanding of the new classification system for periodontitis, readers are directed to the consensus report and case definition paper on periodontitis.

Furthermore, the revised classification now encompasses systemic diseases and conditions affecting the periodontal supporting tissues. Rare systemic disorders, like Papillon-Lefèvre Syndrome, often present with severe early-onset periodontitis and are classified under "Periodontitis as a Manifestation of Systemic Disease," categorized by the primary systemic condition. Other systemic conditions, such as neoplastic diseases, may affect the periodontal tissues independent of plaque-induced periodontitis and are classified based on the primary systemic disease under "Systemic Diseases or Conditions Affecting the Periodontal Supporting Tissues." Common modifiers of periodontitis, like uncontrolled diabetes mellitus, are acknowledged within the new clinical classification as descriptors in the staging and grading process, acknowledging their potential impact on disease progression and treatment outcomes.

The new classification system also introduces revised case definitions for the treatment of gingival recession, incorporating interproximal clinical attachment loss assessments and evaluation of the exposed root and cementoenamel junction. Additionally, a new classification of gingival recession is proposed, integrating clinical parameters such as gingival phenotype and exposed root characteristics. The term "periodontal biotype" has been replaced with "periodontal phenotype" in this context.

Traumatic occlusal force, now referred to as traumatic occlusion, is defined as force exceeding the adaptive capacity of the periodontium and/or teeth, potentially resulting in occlusal trauma, tooth wear. or fracture. While evidence supporting occlusal trauma as a factor in periodontal attachment loss is limited, the terminology has been updated to reflect current understanding.

The section addressing prostheses-related factors has been expanded, with the term "biologic width" replaced by "supracrestal attached tissues." Additionally, clinical procedures involved in indirect restorations have been included, given emerging evidence suggesting their potential impact on recession and clinical attachment loss.

A new classification for peri-implant health, peri-implant mucositis, and peri-implantitis has been developed, aiming for consensus acceptance worldwide. Peri-implant health is defined both clinically and histologically, characterized by the absence of visual signs of inflammation and bleeding on probing. Peri-implant mucositis, on the other hand, presents with bleeding on probing and visual signs of inflammation, with plaque identified as the primary etiological factor. Peri-implantitis, characterized by inflammation and progressive loss of supporting bone, is assumed to follow peri-implant mucositis and is associated with poor plaque control and a history of severe periodontitis. The onset of peri-implantitis may occur early following implant placement, with evidence suggesting a nonlinear and accelerating disease progression in its absence of treatment.

In conclusion, the updated classification system for periodontal and peri-implant diseases and conditions represents a collaborative effort to incorporate contemporary knowledge and clinical practices. It provides a more comprehensive framework for diagnosis, treatment planning, and monitoring, thereby enhancing patient care and outcomes.

3. Periodontal microflora

Periodontal disease, characterized by inflammation and destruction of periodontal tissues, has long been recognized as a multifactorial condition influenced by microbial, genetic, immunological, and environmental factors. Over time, the understanding of periodontal microbiota has undergone significant evolution, transitioning from a simplistic view centered on individual pathogenic bacteria to a more intricate appreciation of microbial communities and their collective impact within biofilms.

The seminal work of Socransky et al. in 1998 introduced the concept of the "red complex," comprising *Porphyromonas gingivalis*, *Treponema denticola*, and *Tannerella forsythia*, as a potent periopathogenic complex associated with severe periodontal disease [2]. Furthermore, *Actinomyces actinomycetemcomitans*, particularly the highly pathogenic JP2 clone, was identified as a significant contributor to aggressive periodontitis, especially in younger individuals [3, 4].

However, recent research has illuminated the intricate interplay between microbial dysbiosis and host response in periodontal disease pathogenesis. The "Inflammation-Mediated Polymicrobial-Emergence and Dysbiotic Exacerbation (IMPEDE)" model has emerged as a novel framework, highlighting the role of dysbiotic plaque biofilms in susceptible hosts in initiating and exacerbating periodontal disease [4].

In addition to the well-known pathogens, several newly identified bacterial species have been implicated in periodontal disease progression [5]. Here are a few recent findings:

Fretibacterium fastidiosum: this is a relatively newly discovered bacterium found in the oral cavity, particularly in individuals with periodontitis. Studies suggest that it may contribute to the progression of periodontal disease by forming biofilms and inducing inflammation [6].

Prevotella histicola: another bacterium associated with periodontitis, *Prevotella histicola* has been found in higher abundance in patients with periodontal disease compared to healthy individuals. It is believed to be involved in the dysbiosis (microbial imbalance), characteristic of periodontitis [7].

Desulfobulbus oralis: this bacterium has been identified as a potential contributor to periodontal disease. Research suggests that it may play a role in the metabolism of sulfur compounds, which could impact the microbial ecology within periodontal pockets [8].

Prevotella pleuritidis: another member of the *Prevotella* genus, *Prevotella pleuritidis* has been found in periodontal pockets of patients with periodontitis. Its specific role in the disease process is still under investigation [9].

In conclusion, the evolution of our understanding of periodontal microflora has shifted the focus from singular pathogenic species to the complex interactions within biofilms and the host immune response. This nuanced perspective emphasizes the importance of considering microbial communities as a whole in periodontal disease etiology and highlights the potential for targeted therapeutic interventions aimed at modulating dysbiosis and mitigating inflammatory processes.

4. Single nucleotide polymorphisms

The hypothesis suggesting the existence of a "high-risk" population group susceptible to periodontitis emerged from seminal clinical research conducted decades ago, which identified varying degrees of disease susceptibility and severity among individuals within the same population [10, 11]. A pivotal study in 1966, examining the primary causes of tooth loss in 1800 patients, revealed a disproportionate number of teeth lost due to periodontitis among a select subset of individuals within each age cohort [12]. This observation was further corroborated by a longitudinal study spanning 28 years, which demonstrated that a small percentage of individuals accounted for a significant majority of total tooth loss during the study period [13].

Chronic periodontitis, the most prevalent form historically, now reclassified into various stages and grades based on severity and risk of progression in the 2018 periodontal disease classification, affects a considerable proportion of adults and typically exhibits a slow progression rate. However, a minority of the population experiences severe forms of periodontitis characterized by rapid tissue destruction, comprising no more than 20% of individuals, constituting the "high-risk group" for the disease. Conversely, most individuals show moderate disease progression, while a small segment exhibits minimal periodontal destruction progression.

In addition to chronic periodontitis, another form known as aggressive periodontitis (now classified as grade C periodontitis) presents with a distinct clinical phenotype characterized by rapid progression and early onset, particularly observed in young, systemically healthy individuals. Within this category, a subgroup known as localized periodontitis grade C, with an incisor-molar pattern, stands out due to its unique clinical presentation, higher prevalence among individuals of African descent, and familial aggregation pattern.

Much of the evidence supporting the role of genetic factors in periodontitis stems from studies focusing on aggressive periodontitis. Observations of increased disease incidence within families, with up to a 50% chance of affected individuals coexisting, underscore the genetic predisposition to this form of the disease. Furthermore, variations in disease prevalence among different racial groups have been noted, with Caucasians exhibiting lower rates compared to individuals of African descent.

Until the early 2000s, investigations into the genetic basis of periodontitis primarily relied on candidate gene approaches, targeting genes implicated in known pathophysiological pathways of the disease. However, this method was limited by the necessity for a priori hypotheses and functional variants in selected genes. As a result, many loci and genes potentially influencing disease susceptibility were overlooked due to limited understanding or involvement in unidentified pathways.

In recent years, genome-wide association studies (GWAS) have revolutionized the study of genetic variants associated with periodontitis. Unlike candidate gene approaches, GWAS offer an unbiased, hypothesis-free approach to screening for disease-associated genetic variants. By simultaneously analyzing millions of single nucleotide polymorphisms (SNPs) across the entire genome, GWAS provide a comprehensive view of genetic contributions to disease susceptibility. SNP, or single nucleotide polymorphism, is a type of genetic variation that occurs within a population. It refers to the variation in a single nucleotide base (A, T, C or G) at a particular position in the DNA sequence among individuals within a species. SNPs are the most common type of genetic variation found in the human genome, with an average occurrence of once every 300 nucleotides. These variations can have an impact on various traits and disease predispositions, which makes them an essential focus of research in genetics, evolutionary biology, and personalized medicine [14].

Modern genetic tools have identified several polymorphisms in genes regulating immune responses and other biological pathways implicated in periodontitis. Among the genes/loci with clear evidence of association with chronic and aggressive periodontitis are Il-1b, Il-1a, MMPs COX2, GLT6D1, ANRIL, DEFB1, IL-10, 25(OH)D metabolites, SIGLEC5, DEFA1A3, MTND1P5, and LOC107984137. Importantly, these genetic associations enhance our understanding of periodontal disease pathogenesis and offer potential avenues for innovative risk assessment, outcome prediction, disease management, and treatment strategies [15–18].

The identification of specific genetic variants associated with periodontitis through GWAS studies offers promising opportunities for translating genetic insights into clinical practice. Incorporating genetic risk assessments into routine periodontal evaluations can enable personalized treatment approaches, including targeted preventive strategies, early intervention for high-risk individuals, and optimized treatment plans tailored to individual genetic profiles. Furthermore, ongoing research in this field holds the potential to develop novel therapeutic interventions aimed at modulating genetic factors implicated in periodontal disease susceptibility, ultimately improving patient outcomes and advancing precision dentistry.

5. Markers of disease activity

Gingival crevicular fluid (GCF) serves as a vital physiological fluid and inflammatory exudate originating from the gingival plexus of blood vessels in the gingival corium, below the epithelium lining of the dentogingival space. Its noninvasive collection from the gingival crevice or periodontal pocket makes it a valuable source for biomarkers associated with periodontal diseases. Collection methods, such as using filter paper or glass capillaries, allow for easy and discomfort-free sampling.

The composition of GCF varies between healthy individuals and those with periodontal diseases, as well as during disease progression. It contains serum-derived components and locally generated biomarkers, offering insights into tissue metabolism, inflammatory cell recruitment, and connective tissue remodeling. GCF reflects the host response to oral microorganisms and the mechanisms by which periodontopathogens exploit these responses for bacterial survival [19].

Proinflammatory cytokines, such as tumor necrosis factor-alpha (TNF-α), interleukin-1α (IL-1α), interleukin-1β (IL-1β), interleukin-6 (IL-6), and interleukin-8 (IL-8), along with metalloproteinases like MMP-8 and MMP-9 [20], are key mediators studied in GCF. These cytokines are products of the innate immune response against bacterial pathogens, contributing to tissue destruction. MMPs, particularly MMP-8, MMP-9, and MMP-13, play crucial roles in extracellular matrix degradation and are implicated in periodontal tissue destruction [21].

Moreover, GCF analysis extends to biochemical markers for bone homeostasis, including pyridinoline cross-linked carboxyterminal telopeptide of type I collagen (ICTP), receptor activator of nuclear factor-kappa β ligand (RANKL), osteoprotegerin (OPG), and osteocalcin. These markers offer insights into future alveolar bone loss prediction and demonstrate significant correlations with clinical parameters and periodontal pathogens.

While single-candidate protein immunoassays have provided valuable insights, they may not offer comprehensive diagnostic support for early periodontal disease. Multiplex protein arrays and mass spectrometry-based proteomics have emerged as promising approaches to characterize the complex network of molecules in GCF. These advanced techniques allow for the identification of novel biomarkers and provide a deeper understanding of disease pathogenesis.

Multiplex protein arrays enable the simultaneous detection and quantification of multiple proteins in GCF, offering a more comprehensive view of the molecular landscape associated with periodontal diseases. This approach allows researchers to examine the interactions between different biomarkers and identify patterns that may be indicative of disease progression or treatment response.

Mass spectrometry-based proteomics offers unparalleled sensitivity and specificity in detecting and quantifying proteins in GCF. By analyzing the entire proteome present in GCF, researchers can uncover novel biomarkers and gain insights into the underlying mechanisms of periodontal diseases [22]. This approach holds great promise for identifying diagnostic and prognostic markers that can aid in personalized treatment strategies.

Overall, proteomic analyses of GCF hold great promise for personalized prevention, diagnosis, and management of periodontal diseases. By complementing clinical examinations, proteomic approaches may enhance our ability to detect and monitor disease activity, ultimately improving patient care outcomes. Continued advancements in proteomic technologies and the exploration of GCF protein profiles offer opportunities for a deeper understanding of periodontal diseases and the development of targeted therapeutic interventions. In the future, integration of proteomic data into clinical practice may enable more precise risk assessment, early detection of disease onset, and personalized treatment planning, leading to improved outcomes for patients with periodontal diseases.

6. Treatment of peri-implantitis

The management of peri-implantitis has evolved alongside advancements in our understanding of peri-implant diseases, with updated guidelines providing comprehensive recommendations for prevention and treatment. Notably, the European Federation of Periodontology (EFP) published a rigorous S3 level Clinical Practice Guideline (CPG) in 2023 [23], following stringent methodological standards set by the Association of Scientific Medical Societies in Germany and utilizing the Grading of Recommendations Assessment, Development, and Evaluation process. This authoritative guideline synthesizes evidence from 13 systematically reviewed studies, evaluates the strength and quality of evidence, and formulates specific recommendations through a consensus process involving leading experts and stakeholders.

These guidelines serve as a pivotal resource for clinicians, healthcare systems, policymakers, and the public, offering evidence-based strategies spanning pre-, peri-, and post-implant phases to mitigate peri-implant diseases. Notably, the focus lies on preventive measures, commencing with primordial prevention strategies aimed at modulating lifestyle and behavioral risk factors, coupled with meticulous surgical and prosthetic planning to preempt the onset of peri-implant mucositis and peri-implantitis.

In the management of peri-implant diseases, the guideline delineates distinct treatment modalities tailored to specific phases and objectives. For instance, in addressing peri-implant mucositis, interventions primarily emphasize effective self-administered oral hygiene and professional mechanical plaque removal (PMPR), while pharmacotherapeutic interventions like photodynamic therapy and systemic/local antibiotics are cautioned against. Furthermore, the guideline highlights the potential benefits of adjunctive oral rinse antiseptics alongside PMPR for a limited duration.

Conversely, the management of peri-implantitis encompasses both non-surgical and surgical interventions, often adopting a stepwise approach. The non-surgical phase aims to control peri-implant biofilms and inflammation through techniques such as sub-marginal instrumentation, supplemented by strategies targeting supra-marginal biofilm control and risk factor management. Despite the lack of established endpoints akin to periodontitis treatment, vigilant monitoring and reassessment of outcomes remain integral.

In cases where non-surgical interventions fall short of desired outcomes, surgical intervention becomes imperative. Surgical procedures typically involve flap elevation, removal of inflamed tissue, decontamination of implant surfaces, and, where necessary, reconstructive approaches to manage peri-implant osseous defects. The guideline also underscores the potential role of adjunctive measures such as implant surface decontamination and local/systemic antibiotics.

Overall, the stepwise approach advocated by the guideline underscores the importance of optimizing biofilm and inflammation control before considering more invasive interventions. While further research is warranted to refine treatment protocols and establish definitive endpoints, adherence to evidence-based guidelines ensures the delivery of optimal care and improved outcomes for patients with peri-implant diseases.

In summary, the guidelines established by the European Federation of Periodontology (EFP) offer a comprehensive approach to the prevention and treatment of peri-implant diseases. By integrating the latest research and employing a rigorous methodology, these guidelines provide clinicians with standardized strategies for addressing peri-implant mucositis and peri-implantitis. Key components of these guidelines include primordial prevention strategies targeting lifestyle and behavioral risk factors, as well as meticulous surgical and prosthetic planning to mitigate disease development. Treatment approaches are tailored to specific phases and objectives, with a focus on optimizing biofilm and inflammation control before considering surgical interventions. Looking ahead, the adoption of these guidelines is expected to usher in a new era of precision dentistry, where treatment approaches are personalized based on individual patient needs and risk profiles. By adhering to evidence-based guidelines, clinicians can enhance treatment outcomes and improve the longevity of dental implants, ultimately shaping the future of clinical practice in peri-implant dentistry.

7. Guided dental implant placement

Guided (computed) dental implant surgery was first introduced in late 1990s and since then was evolved due to recent development of digital technology to an easier and more accurate guided dental implant placement, ideal both prosthetically and biologically [24].

Guided dental implant placement has been classified recently into partial or full guidance and the ability to make intraoperative changes before implant placement named either static or dynamic guided implant placement. Recently guided implant surgery has been developed to be applied in a flapless procedure.

Taking into consideration that cone beam computed tomography is a highly accurate and low radiation tomography, the application of flapless guided implant surgery has become very popular. Studies have shown that it has lower morbidity, as it is less invasive, compared to flapped approach. This technique should be limited to cases that do not need bone augmentation and have a wide zone of keratinized tissue. Both flapped and flapless guided implant surgery might show some inaccuracies with respect to the planned implant position.

According to metanalytic measures of dispersions, safety margins should always be applied. A safety margin of 2 mm in depth and 2–3 mm in coronoapical bodily position and 4° angulation should be followed in order to avoid postsurgical implications.

The development and use of navigation systems for dental implant placement has inspired surgeons to investigate the field of robot-assisted implant surgery. Visual, audio, and haptic feedbacks are used in real time to position the implant drill in the correct 3D location. The surgeon could only move the arm which carries the handpiece closer toward the correct position. As the precision of the implant placement is high and allows prefabrication of the prosthesis, most of dental implants can be loaded immediately, if biological factors such as bone quality allow it [25, 26].

Overall, recent advances in dental implant placement technology have made dental implant placement more accurate, with less morbidity and less invasive. These innovations hold promise for improving patient outcomes and expanding the possibilities of implant dentistry.

8. Teeth or dental implants or mesenchymal cells that can grow a tooth

Treatment and long-term preservation of periodontally compromised teeth have always posed significant challenges in dental practice. Moreover, rehabilitating partially or fully edentulous periodontal patients has been notably complex, particularly before the advent of dental implants as a viable treatment option. In cases of advanced periodontal disease, clinicians must meticulously evaluate clinical and radiographic findings alongside tooth and patient-related risk factors [27].

Various publications have proposed different algorithms and criteria for assessing the prognosis of periodontally compromised teeth. For instance, McGuire and Nunn categorized teeth with Class II or III furcation involvement and substantial attachment loss resulting in a poor crown-to-root ratio as 'questionable', while designating a tooth as 'hopeless' if the remaining clinical attachment level is insufficient to maintain health, comfort, and function, thus necessitating extraction before comprehensive mouth rehabilitation.

Fortunately, the emergence of dental implant dentistry has provided clinicians with a successful and predictable alternative for addressing complete or partial edentulism. The inclusion of dental implants in the treatment of periodontal patients with missing teeth has been well-established, with multiple longitudinal studies demonstrating highly satisfactory results in terms of both survival and success rates. A recent systematic review by Sousa et al. [28] highlighted implant survival rates of 88–98.8% and 92.4–100% over 5–10 years in patients with moderate and advanced periodontal disease, respectively [29].

However, it is crucial to acknowledge the common etiology shared between periodontal and peri-implant diseases, with peri-implantitis and perimucositis being prevalent in patients with a history of periodontal disease. This complicates the rehabilitation of periodontal patients with dental implants, as lesions around implants tend to exhibit a more destructive inflammatory profile and faster progression compared to periodontitis. Furthermore, biofilm removal from implant surfaces can be more challenging due to surface roughness and macro-design, as opposed to dental implant surfaces.

In recent years, medicine has increasingly focused on regenerative approaches employing pluripotent mesenchymal cells. Within dentistry, tissue engineering offers several avenues, including the utilization of stem cells. Specifically, for the regeneration of periodontal tissues, a robust blood supply is essential, as it facilitates the transport of necessary molecules for regeneration. Dental pulp mesenchymal stem cells (DP-MSCs) have shown promise in inducing neoangiogenesis, followed by the formation of a vascular network in the periodontal niche. Additionally, research suggests that DP-MSCs derived from deciduous teeth can differentiate into functional dentin, cementum, and periodontal ligament tissues, including bone.

In conclusion, DP-MSCs hold significant potential for future applications in treating periodontitis and, importantly, for regenerating periodontal tissues without adverse reactions. Continued research and advancements in this area may lead to transformative therapeutic options for managing periodontal disease and enhancing patient outcomes.

9. Probiotics and vaccines

Effective prevention and treatment of the most common oral diseases, including gingivitis, periodontitis, and caries, require collaborative efforts between patients and oral health specialists [30]. While bacterial plaque accumulation in the periodontal environment is a primary driver of periodontal diseases, various host response factors significantly influence disease progression. These factors, encompassing aspects of innate and adaptive immunity, polymorphonuclear neutrophil function, upregulation of pro-inflammatory cytokines, matrix metalloproteinases, and wound healing properties, collectively modulate the progression and severity of periodontal diseases among individuals [31].

In response to the complex interplay of microbial and host factors in periodontal disease pathogenesis, novel approaches targeting inflammation control and immunomodulation have emerged. Probiotics and oral vaccines represent two such innovative strategies for the prevention and treatment of periodontal diseases [32].

Probiotics, defined by the Food and Agricultural Organization/World Health Organization as live microorganisms that, when administered in adequate amounts, confer health benefits to the host and offer promising avenues for periodontal disease prevention [33]. Mechanisms underlying the beneficial effects of probiotics in preventing periodontal disease include the reversal of damage to oral epithelia and mucosa caused by inflammation, modulation of the oral microbiota by competing with dysbiotic microflora for resources, and production of antimicrobial factors that inhibit the proliferation of gram-negative bacteria [32]. While the potential of probiotics to modulate the oral microbiota and exert immune-modulatory effects is promising, further research is needed to identify the most effective probiotic strains for maintaining oral health and to demonstrate their clinical efficacy [34].

Another innovative approach involves the development of oral mucosa-administered vaccines targeting specific pathogens implicated in periodontal disease pathogenesis, such as *Porphyromonas gingivalis*, *Tannerella forsythia*, and *Treponema denticola* [31]. These Gram-negative anaerobic bacteria produce virulence factors that stimulate the host immune response, making them ideal vaccine targets. Proposed vaccines include those targeting whole-cell antigens, gingipains, fimbriae, and other virulence factors of periodontal pathogens. While the development of periodontal vaccines holds promise, additional studies are needed to establish their clinical efficacy in human models.

In conclusion, probiotics and oral vaccines represent innovative approaches in the prevention and treatment of periodontal diseases. Continued research efforts are essential to elucidate their mechanisms of action, identify optimal formulations and dosages, and validate their clinical effectiveness. Additionally, ongoing exploration of other novel strategies, such as antimicrobial peptides, host modulation therapy, and personalized medicine, holds promise for further enhancing our ability to combat periodontal diseases effectively in the future.

10. Minimally invasive surgery

In the realm of periodontal therapy, the evolution toward minimally invasive surgical (MIS) techniques marks a significant stride in enhancing treatment precision while prioritizing patient comfort and aesthetic outcomes. These approaches, meticulously crafted to preserve soft tissues and achieve stable primary wound closure, stand as pivotal advancements in modern periodontal care [35].

The integration of operating microscopes and microsurgical instruments has revolutionized surgical precision, offering enhanced visual capacity and refined control over surgical maneuvers while minimizing tissue disruption [36]. The inception of MIS in 1995 heralded a new era in periodontal surgery, with its core tenets centered around minimizing wounds, flap reflection, and trauma to surrounding tissues [37]. Subsequent reports underscore the clinical efficacy of MIS, showcasing improvements in key parameters such as probing pocket depth reduction and clinical attachment level gain [38].

A notable refinement in MIS is the minimally invasive surgical technique (MIST), tailored specifically for treating isolated intra-bony defects with a focus on periodontal regeneration. This technique, integrating established papilla preservation strategies and meticulous suturing, not only reduces surgical trauma but also ensures stable wound closure and enhanced patient comfort [39].

Building upon these foundations, the modified minimally invasive surgical technique (M-MIST) further refines surgical invasiveness by preserving the interdental papilla while raising only a buccal flap, thereby optimizing esthetic outcomes and tissue healing [40]. Recent advancements have introduced innovative techniques such as the single flap approach (SFA), connective tissue graft wall technique, non-incised papilla surgical approach, and modified vestibular incision subperiosteal tunnel access (M-VISTA).

The SFA, characterized by the elevation of a mucoperiosteal flap on one side while preserving soft tissues on the opposite side, exemplifies the pursuit of optimal esthetic outcomes [41]. Similarly, the connective tissue graft wall technique, coupled with enamel matrix derivative, presents a formidable approach for treating deep vertical bony defects and associated gingival recession [42].

In alignment with the ethos of minimally invasive surgery, the non-incised papilla surgical approach and M-VISTA prioritize tissue preservation and esthetic integrity by minimizing trauma to marginal tissues and avoiding unnecessary incisions [43, 44].

Moreover, the minimal access flap (MAF) technique and closed surgical technique (CST) exemplify the commitment to minimally invasive principles by retaining tissue integrity and promoting regeneration while minimizing patient discomfort [45].

In summary, the relentless pursuit of precision and patient-centric care underscores the ongoing evolution of minimally invasive surgical approaches in periodontics. By amalgamating cutting-edge techniques with a steadfast commitment to optimal outcomes, MIS stands as a beacon of innovation in modern periodontal therapy.

11. Advances in perio-ortho treatment

Patients grappling with periodontitis often necessitate an interdisciplinary approach that includes orthodontic intervention to effectively restore masticatory function, aesthetics, and overall quality of life. Progressive loss of periodontal tissues can lead to tooth drifting, flaring, secondary occlusal trauma, bite collapse, masticatory dysfunction, and ultimately tooth loss [46]. These considerations are integral to the newly introduced Classification of Periodontal and Peri-implant Diseases, where they serve as diagnostic criteria for stage IV, representing the most severe form of periodontitis. Guidelines published by the European Federation of Periodontology provide detailed insights into the timing of orthodontic treatment (OT) in periodontally compromised patients. It is recommended to commence OT only once the endpoints of periodontal therapy have been met, typically characterized by the absence of sites with probing pocket depth (PPD) ≤ 5 mm and positive bleeding on probing (BOP), along with the absence of sites with PPD ≥ 6 mm. These endpoints are usually achieved following non-surgical or surgical periodontal therapy as deemed necessary [47].

For teeth with intrabony defects, OT can be initiated soon after surgical treatment, as this combined approach has demonstrated favorable clinical outcomes and enhances the long-term prognosis of severely periodontally compromised teeth [48, 49]. Incisors afflicted with bone loss are particularly susceptible to elongation owing to the absence of occlusal and anteroposterior contacts. In cases of severe tooth loss inhibiting vertical migration during orthodontic correction, intrusion and retraction maneuvers are often necessary. Circumferential supracrestal fibrotomy, repeated monthly during intrusive movement, may reduce marginal bone resorption and facilitate these corrective movements.

Addressing gingival recession therapy, situations where the root is in close proximity to or beyond the cortical bone may benefit from orthodontic repositioning of the root within the bone prior to surgical root coverage procedures. Clear aligners, alongside traditional brackets, serve as effective tools for repositioning lower incisors' roots before surgical root coverage procedures [50]. Moreover, periodontal phenotype modification therapy (PhMT), encompassing hard tissue augmentation (PhMT-b) or soft tissue augmentation (PhMT-s), prior to OT initiation could prevent loss of periodontal support and gingival recession, particularly in patients with thin and scalloped phenotypes [51].

Lastly, the latest advancements in combined periodontal and orthodontic treatment include the utilization of osseointegrated implants as orthodontic anchorage. These implants offer superior orthodontic anchorage compared to traditional tooth-borne devices, particularly beneficial in cases of inadequate periodontal anchorage, patient non-compliance with anchorage aids, aesthetic concerns or the desire to avoid post-growth completion orthognathic surgery [52].

These advancements underscore the evolving landscape of periodontal-orthodontic treatment, where integrated approaches hold immense potential for optimizing patient outcomes and overall treatment efficacy.

12. Biomaterials for periodontal regeneration

Periodontal therapy aims at achieving new periodontal attachment formation, making guided tissue regeneration (GTR) a pivotal surgical technique [53]. Barrier biomaterials play a crucial role by physically impeding fast-growing soft tissue cells like epithelial cells and gingival fibroblasts from infiltrating defective sites during periodontal regeneration. While the initial GTR membranes utilized non-resorbable materials, such as expanded polytetrafluoroethylene, the advent of resorbable membranes like collagen addressed the need for membrane removal surgeries. Recent decades have witnessed the development of membranes from synthetic polymers and naturally derived sources like collagen-based, chitosan, alginate, as well as occlusive titanium and micro-perforated titanium membranes. Additionally, advancements in tissue engineering and the integration of drug delivery systems into membranes hold promise for enhancing the barrier concept associated with guided bone regeneration (GBR) [54].

To achieve periodontal regeneration and alveolar ridge reconstruction, graft materials are commonly employed in conjunction with barrier membranes. These materials encompass autografts, allografts, xenografts, and alloplastic materials. While conventional biomaterials remain primary sources for periodontal regeneration, recent years have seen the development of new biomaterials for cementum, periodontal ligament (PDL), and alveolar bone regeneration. Ceramic biomaterials like calcium phosphate (CaP), calcium sulfate (CS), and bioactive glass (BG) exhibit characteristics conducive to hard tissue engineering due to their composition similar to bone mineral and their capacity to stimulate cell proliferation and differentiation [55]. With the emergence of tissue engineering and additive manufacturing, novel approaches like cell sheet engineering and multiphasic scaffolds have surfaced, with current research focusing on regenerating cementum, PDL, or the entire periodontium [56]. Furthermore, 3D printing facilitates the creation of precise scaffolds with controlled shape and porosity, with biomimetic 3D printing scaffolds being developed for regenerating complex alveolar bone-PDL-cementum structures [53].

A recent approach revolves around employing bioactive agents (BAs) to treat intra-osseous and furcation defects in conjunction with grafts and/or GTR. BAs such as recombinant human platelet-derived growth factor-BB (rhPDGF-BB), fibroblast growth factor (FGF), insulin-like growth factor (IGF), bone morphogenetic proteins (BMPs), platelet-rich plasma (PRP), enamel matrix derivative (EMD), and peptide P-15 (P-15) have been clinically evaluated for treating periodontal defects [41]. EMD and PRP products have garnered considerable interest and are widely utilized for periodontal regeneration. EMD, for instance, has demonstrated efficacy in intrabony defects, particularly when coupled with minimally invasive surgical techniques or flapless techniques, thereby enhancing initial wound stability and minimizing patient morbidity. Moreover, EMD has shown promise in recession defects, both alone and as an adjunct to soft tissue grafting, as well as in furcation defects [57]. Looking ahead, EMD's applications are expanding to include supraalveolar-type defects with access flap surgery and possibly the treatment of peri-implantitis and mucosal recessions around implants [58].

Clinical research suggests that combined therapy involving platelet-rich plasma (PRP) with bone grafts and/or cells holds potential for ridge augmentation procedures. However, further randomized controlled trials (RCTs) are necessary to ascertain the superiority of specific autologous platelet concentrates (APCs). While APCs may expedite clinical healing, soft tissue epithelialization, and reduce postoperative pain in ridge preservation procedures, evidence regarding their significant impact on hard tissue regeneration remains inconclusive [54].

These advancements underscore a promising trajectory in the field of periodontal regeneration, with ongoing research poised to drive further innovation and clinical application.

13. Conclusions

In recent years, both medicine and dentistry have experienced significant advancements. Within dentistry, particularly in periodontology, there has been a rapid evolution in research and clinical approaches. This evolution spans various aspects, including prevention, diagnosis, prognosis, and treatment of periodontal diseases. Notably, there has been a shift toward prioritizing patient satisfaction by adopting less-invasive therapeutic approaches and emphasizing regeneration techniques aimed at restoring the original architecture of periodontal tissues.

Furthermore, innovations in antibiotic-probiotic treatment modalities have emerged, leveraging insights from the exploration of new bacteria and biofilm construction. This enhanced understanding has paved the way for more personalized periodontal treatment strategies tailored to individual genetic factors. Additionally, the introduction of robotic surgical techniques holds promise for minimizing trauma and enhancing surgical precision in periodontal interventions.

Overall, these advancements reflect a concerted effort within the field of periodontology to embrace cutting-edge technologies and evidence-based practices, ultimately aiming to improve patient outcomes and quality of care.

Author details

Neophytou Chariklia, Kolovou Stolina, Konstantinos Papadimitriou and Aikaterini-Elisavet Doufexi*
Department of Preventive Dentistry, Periodontology and Implant Biology, School of Dentistry, Aristotle University of Thessaloniki, Greece

*Address all correspondence to: doufexi@dent.auth.gr

References

[1] Caton JG, Armitage G, Berglundh T, Chapple ILC, Jepsen S, Kornman KS, et al. A new classification scheme for periodontal and peri-implant diseases and conditions – Introduction and key changes from the 1999 classification. Journal of Clinical Periodontology. 2018;**45**(S20):159-172

[2] Socransky SS, Haffajee AD, Cugini MA, Smith C, Kent RL. Microbial complexes in subgingival plaque. Journal of Clinical Periodontology. 1998;**25**(2):134-144

[3] Armitage GC. Development of a Classification System for Periodontal Diseases and Conditions. Annals of Periodontology. 1999;**4**(1):1-6

[4] Mehta J, Eaton C, AlAmri M, Lin G, Nibali L. The association between *Aggregatibacter actinomycetemcomitans* JP2 clone and periodontitis: A systematic review and meta-analysis. Journal of Periodontal Research. 2023;**58**(3):465-482

[5] Jusko M, Miedziak B, Ermert D, Magda M, King BC, Bielecka E, et al. FACIN, a double-edged sword of the emerging periodontal pathogen *Filifactor alocis*: A metabolic enzyme moonlighting as a complement inhibitor. The Journal of Immunology. 2016;**197**(8):3245-3259

[6] Oliveira RRDS, Fermiano D, Feres M, Figueiredo LC, Teles FRF, Soares GMS, et al. Levels of candidate periodontal pathogens in subgingival biofilm. Journal of Dental Research. 2016;**95**(6):711-718

[7] Downes J, Hooper SJ, Wilson MJ, Wade WG. Prevotella histicola sp. nov., isolated from the human oral cavity. International Journal of Systematic and Evolutionary Microbiology. 2008;**58**(8):1788-1791

[8] Castillo Y, Delgadillo NA, Neuta Y, Iniesta M, Sanz M, Herrera D, et al. Design and validation of a quantitative polymerase chain reaction test for the identification and quantification of uncultivable bacteria associated with periodontitis. Archives of Oral Biology. 2023;**154**:105758

[9] Esberg A, Johansson L, Johansson I, Dahlqvist SR. Oral microbiota identifies patients in early onset rheumatoid arthritis. Microorganisms. 2021;**9**(8):1657

[10] Löe H, Anerud A, Boysen H, Morrison E. Natural history of periodontal disease in man. Journal of Clinical Periodontology. 1986;**13**(5):431-440

[11] Schätzle M, Löe H, Lang NP, Heitz-Mayfield LJA, Bürgin W, Ånerud Å, et al. Clinical course of chronic periodontitis. Journal of Clinical Periodontology. 2003;**30**(10):909-918

[12] Trott JR, Cross HG. An analysis of the principle reasons for tooth extractions in 1813 patients in Manitoba. The Dental Practitioner and Dental Record. 1966;**17**(1):20-27

[13] Hirschfeld L, Wasserman B. A long-term survey of tooth loss in 600 treated periodontal patients. Journal of Periodontology. 1978;**49**(5):225-237

[14] The international hapmap consortium. The International HapMap Project. Nature. 2003;**426**(6968):789-796

[15] Offenbacher S, Divaris K, Barros SP, Moss KL, Marchesan JT, Morelli T, et al. Genome-wide association study of biologically informed periodontal complex traits offers novel insights into the genetic basis of periodontal disease. Human Molecular Genetics. 2016;**25**(10):2113-2129

[16] Divaris K, Monda KL, North KE, Olshan AF, Lange EM, Moss K, et al. Genome-wide association study of periodontal pathogen colonization. Journal of Dental Research. 2012;**91**(7_suppl):S21-S28

[17] Schaefer AS, Richter GM, Nothnagel M, Manke T, Dommisch H, Jacobs G, et al. A genome-wide association study identifies GLT6D1 as a susceptibility locus for periodontitis. Human Molecular Genetics. 2010;**19**(3):553-562

[18] Munz M, Richter GM, Loos BG, Jepsen S, Divaris K, Offenbacher S, et al. Meta-analysis of genome-wide association studies of aggressive and chronic periodontitis identifies two novel risk loci. European Journal of Human Genetics. 2019;**27**(1):102-113

[19] Barros SP, Williams R, Offenbacher S, Morelli T. Gingival crevicular fluid as a source of biomarkers for periodontitis. Periodontology 2000. 2000;**70**(1):53-64

[20] Luchian I, Goriuc A, Sandu D, Covasa M. The role of matrix metalloproteinases (MMP-8, MMP-9, MMP-13) in periodontal and peri-implant pathological processes. International Journal of Molecular Sciences. 2022;**23**(3):1806

[21] Zhang Z, Yang X, Zhang H, Liu X, Pan S, Li C. The role of extracellular matrix metalloproteinase inducer glycosylation in regulating matrix metalloproteinases in periodontitis. Journal of Periodontal Research. 2018;**53**(3):391-402

[22] Guzman YA, Sakellari D, Arsenakis M, Floudas CA. Proteomics for the discovery of biomarkers and diagnosis of periodontitis: A critical review. Expert Review of Proteomics. 2014;**11**(1):31-41

[23] Herrera D, Berglundh T, Schwarz F, Chapple I, Jepsen S, Sculean A, et al. Prevention and treatment of peri-implant diseases—The EFP S3 level clinical practice guideline. Journal of Clinical Periodontology. 2023;**50**(S26):4-76

[24] Romandini M, Ruales-Carrera E, Sadilina S, Hämmerle CHF, Sanz M. Minimal invasiveness at dental implant placement: A systematic review with meta-analyses on flapless fully guided surgery. Periodontology 2000. 2000. 2023;**91**(1):89-112

[25] Marlière DAA, Demètrio MS, Picinini LS, De Oliveira RG, Netto HD. Accuracy of computer-guided surgery for dental implant placement in fully edentulous patients: A systematic review. European Journal of Dentistry. 2018;**12**(01):153-160

[26] Naeini EN, Atashkadeh M, De Bruyn H, D'Haese J. Narrative review regarding the applicability, accuracy, and clinical outcome of flapless implant surgery with or without computer guidance. Clinical Implant Dentistry and Related Research. 2020;**22**(4):454-467

[27] Sarafidou K, Lazaridi I, Gotsis S, Kirmanidou Y, Vasilaki D, Hirayama H, et al. Tooth preservation vs. extraction and implant placement in periodontally compromised patients: A systematic review and analysis of studies. Journal of Prosthodontics. 2022;**31**(8):87-99

[28] Sousa V, Mardas N, Farias B, Petrie A, Needleman I, Spratt D, et al. A systematic review of implant outcomes in treated periodontitis patients. Clinical Oral Implants Research. 2016;**27**(7):787-844

[29] Rösing CK, Fiorini T, Haas AN, Muniz FW, Oppermann RV, Susin C. The impact of maintenance on peri-implant

health. Brazilian Oral Research. 2019;**33**(suppl. 1):e74-83

[30] Scannapieco FA, Gershovich E. The prevention of periodontal disease—An overview. Periodontology 2000. 2020;**84**(1):9-13

[31] Sczepanik FSC, Grossi ML, Casati M, Goldberg M, Glogauer M, Fine N, et al. Periodontitis is an inflammatory disease of oxidative stress: We should treat it that way. Periodontology 2000. 2020;**84**(1):45-68

[32] Myneni SR, Brocavich K, Wang H, H. Biological strategies for the prevention of periodontal disease: Probiotics and vaccines. Periodontology 2000. 2020;**84**(1):161-175

[33] Teughels W, Loozen G, Quirynen M. Do probiotics offer opportunities to manipulate the periodontal oral microbiota? Journal of Clinical Periodontology. 2011;**38**(s11):159-177

[34] Tonetti MS, Chapple ILC. Biological approaches to the development of novel periodontal therapies – Consensus of the Seventh European Workshop on Periodontology. Journal of Clinical Periodontology. 2011;**38**(s11):114-118

[35] Cortellini P, Prato GP, Tonetti MS. The modified papilla preservation technique. A New Surgical Approach for Interproximal Regenerative Procedures. Journal of Periodontology. 1995;**66**(4):261-266

[36] Cortellini P, Tonetti MS. Clinical performance of a regenerative strategy for intrabony defects: Scientific evidence and clinical experience. Journal of Periodontology. 2005;**76**(3):341-350

[37] Harrel SK, Rees TD. Granulation tissue removal in routine and minimally invasive procedures. The Compendium of Continuing Education in Dentistry. 1995;**16**(9):960, 962, 964 passim

[38] Harrel SK. A minimally invasive surgical approach for periodontal bone grafting. The International Journal of Periodontics & Restorative Dentistry. 1998;**18**(2):161-169

[39] Cortellini P, Prato GP, Tonetti MS. The simplified papilla preservation flap. A novel surgical approach for the management of soft tissues in regenerative procedures. The International Journal of Periodontics & Restorative Dentistry. 1999;**19**(6):589-599

[40] Cortellini P, Tonetti MS. Improved wound stability with a modified minimally invasive surgical technique in the regenerative treatment of isolated interdental intrabony defects. Journal of Clinical Periodontology. 2009;**36**(2):157-163

[41] Trombelli L, Farina R, Franceschetti G, Calura G. Single-flap approach with buccal access in periodontal reconstructive procedures. Journal of Periodontology. 2009;**80**(2):353-360

[42] Zucchelli G, Marzadori M, Mazzotti C, Felice P, Stefanini M. Connective tissue graft wall technique and enamel matrix derivative for the treatment of infrabony defects: Case reports. The International Journal of Periodontics & Restorative Dentistry. 2017;**37**(5):673-681

[43] Moreno Rodriguez J, Caffesse R. Nonincised papillae surgical approach (NIPSA) in periodontal regeneration: Preliminary results of a case series. The International Journal of Periodontics & Restorative Dentistry. 2018;**38**:s105-s111

[44] Najafi B, Kheirieh P, Torabi A, Cappetta E. Periodontal regenerative treatment of intrabony defects in the

esthetic zone using modified vestibular incision subperiosteal tunnel access (M-VISTA). The International Journal of Periodontics & Restorative Dentistry. 2018;**38**:e9-e16

[45] Apatzidou DA, Bakopoulou AA, Kouzi-Koliakou K, Karagiannis V, Konstantinidis A. A tissue-engineered biocomplex for periodontal reconstruction. A proof-of-principle randomized clinical study. Journal of Clinical Periodontology. 2021;**48**(8):1111-1125

[46] Oruba Z, Gibas-Stanek M, Pihut M, Cześnikiewicz-Guzik M, Stós W. Orthodontic treatment in patients with periodontitis – A narrative literature review. Australian Dental Journal. 2023;**68**(4):238-246

[47] Herrera D, Sanz M, Kebschull M, Jepsen S, Sculean A, Berglundh T, et al. Treatment of stage IV periodontitis: The EFP S3 level clinical practice guideline. Journal of Clinical Periodontology. 2022;**49**(S24):4-71

[48] Sanz M, Herrera D, Kebschull M, Chapple I, Jepsen S, Berglundh T, et al. Treatment of stage I–III periodontitis—The EFP S3 level clinical practice guideline. Journal of Clinical Periodontology. 2020;**47**(S22):4-60

[49] Kloukos D, Roccuzzo A, Stähli A, Sculean A, Katsaros C, Salvi GE. Effect of combined periodontal and orthodontic treatment of tilted molars and of teeth with intra-bony and furcation defects in stage- IV periodontitis patients: A systematic review. Journal of Clinical Periodontology. 2022;**49**(S24):121-148

[50] Chaushu S, Stabholz A. Orthodontic-associated localized gingival recession of lower incisors: Who should treat it? Compendium of Continuing Education in Dentistry. 2013;**34**:6-12; quiz 13

[51] Wang C, Yu S, Mandelaris GA, Wang H. Is periodontal phenotype modification therapy beneficial for patients receiving orthodontic treatment? An American Academy of Periodontology best evidence review. Journal of Periodontology. 2020;**91**(3):299-310

[52] Melsen B, Lang NP. Biological reactions of alveolar bone to orthodontic loading of oral implants. Clinical Oral Implants Research. 2001;**12**(2):144-152

[53] Deng Y, Liang Y, Liu X. Biomaterials for periodontal regeneration. Dental Clinics of North America. 2022;**66**(4):659-672

[54] Sanz M, Dahlin C, Apatzidou D, Artzi Z, Bozic D, Calciolari E, et al. Biomaterials and regenerative technologies used in bone regeneration in the craniomaxillofacial region: Consensus report of group 2 of the 15th European Workshop on Periodontology on Bone Regeneration. Journal of Clinical Periodontology. 2019;**46**(S21):82-91

[55] Snyder AJ, Levin MP, Cutright DE. Alloplastic implants of tricalcium phosphate ceramic in human periodontal osseous defects. Journal of Periodontology. 1984;**55**(5):273-277

[56] Ni C, Zhou J, Kong N, Bian T, Zhang Y, Huang X, et al. Gold nanoparticles modulate the crosstalk between macrophages and periodontal ligament cells for periodontitis treatment. Biomaterials. 2019;**206**:115-132

[57] Miron RJ, Sculean A, Cochran DL, Froum S, Zucchelli G, Nemcovsky C, et al. Twenty years of enamel matrix derivative: The past, the present and the future. Journal of Clinical Periodontology. 2016;**43**(8):668-683

[58] Froum SJ, Froum SH, Rosen PS. Successful management of peri-implantitis with a regenerative approach: A consecutive series of 51 treated implants with 3- to 7.5-year follow-up. The International Journal of Periodontics & Restorative Dentistry. 2012;**32**(1):11-20

Chapter 2

Epigenetics and Stem Cells Applications in Periodontal Therapy

Faten Kafa

Abstract

While periodontitis is closely linked with pathogen outgrowth, many patients have the risk of recurrence after therapy. Variations of inflammatory genes are associated with an increased susceptibility of periodontitis. Epigenetics can regulate these gene expression. In this chapter, we will highlight on the potential role of epigenetic changes in different facets, more particularly in genes involved in inflammation. Epigenetics act through remodeling of chromatin and can selectively activate or inactivate genes, determining their expression. Epigenetics could play an essential role in understanding the mechanism of gene-environment interactions, and the factors which stimulate periodontitis and reduce its response to therapy are now the subject of many studies. Also, mesenchymal stem cells (MSCs) are a promising source to regenerate periodontal tissues. They could be a good alternative to the adopted therapies, ignoring the artificial biomaterial limitations. They could be considered as a natural process for periodontium regeneration and has an immunomodulatory role to resolute the infection. For this reason, it is necessary to investigate and evaluate MSCs applicability in humans, and their clinical approach involved in regeneration of periodontal tissues.

Keywords: epigenetics, periodontitis, stem cells, methylation, histone modifications, new therapeutic approaches

1. Introduction

Periodontitis is a chronic inflammatory disease caused by a gram-negative bacterial plaque located on gingiva and teeth surfaces. It is induced by immune imbalance between the plaque and host inflammatory response toward the alveolar bone [1]. It is frequently encountered in the oral cavity affecting the structures that support teeth, leading to periodontal pocket, loss of attachment, and alveolar remodeling [2, 3].

Periodontitis is a complex disease caused by multiple factors, extrinsic (modifiable), and intrinsic (nonmodifiable) factors [4]. Although its mechanisms are still unclear, outgrowth of multiple opportunistic microbes mainly contributes to inflammation, but it is not solely sufficient factor leading to this condition. Numerous risk factors can impede the immune response and periodontitis prevalence [5], like environmental factors, systemic inflammation diseases such as diabetes [6], cardiovascular diseases [7], metabolic syndrome [8], and pneumonia [9], lifestyle-related factors, such as smoking and diet, as well as oral hygiene [10], and genetic variables [11].

Although most of the periodontal studies have focused on microbial pathogens and oral environments, inflammation susceptibility association with intrinsic factors such as genetics is also determined. Some people are more disease-susceptible or treatment resistant, which emphasizes that fact.

In this chapter, we summarize the most important genetic factors in periodontitis progression and focus on epigenetic modifications involved in the etiology of periodontitis, which can be considered as mediators between environmental and genetic factors. This information could be useful guidelines for new biomarker that will help in periodontitis diagnosis and treatment.

2. Periodontitis-related genetic variation

2.1 SNPs in inflammatory genes

Genetic factors are very important in periodontitis development, but we can consider genetic variations as a risk factor only when combined with external agents and physical activities. Genetic variations associated with multifactorial diseases cannot be able to define easily.

Genetic polymorphisms can be caused by a single nucleotide substitution in a DNA sequence with another one, deletion or insertion one or more nucleotides, or repetitive sequences insertion [12]. The polymorphism leads to a change in the coded protein structure if it occurs in an exon, the part of the gene that codes the protein, while it can lead to a change in gene function if it comes in the non-coding sequence (intron). Changes in the transcription-regulating sequence (promoter) can affect gene expression [12].

Single nucleotide polymorphism (SNP) in a gene is used as a genetic marker when it can express a special phenotype [4]. Periodontitis susceptibility can be detected with a SNP. Many studies have focused on the description of genetic polymorphism effect in inflammatory proteins and gene expression in several populations. They have shown that susceptibility is clearly affected by multiple allelic variants [13].

Defensins (DEFB) are important components of innate immunity and extensively exist in the gingival tissue. SNPs in defensin gene have been detected to correlate with gene expression and with the risk of periodontitis [14]. Pro-inflammatory cytokines have a critical role in periodontitis pathogenesis, and their gene SNPs may influence the degree of host response to microbial infection and then the disease severity [13, 15].

The most periodontitis-related SNPs have been studied in the Toll-like receptor-2 (TLR-2) [16], TLR-4 [17], Fc-γ receptor (FCGR2A) [18], interleukin-1 (IL-1) [19–21], IL-4 [22], IL-6 [23–25], IL-10 [23, 26], IL-18 [27, 28], vitamin D receptor [11, 29], tumor necrosis factor alpha (TNFA) [30–32], matrix metalloproteinase (MMP) [33, 34], and cyclo-oxygenase-2 (COX-2) [35].

These studies have determined the relationship of genetic polymorphisms at multiple loci with periodontitis, but it is still unclear. It should be noted that this relation is not always strong due to differences between populations and periodontitis subtypes.

2.2 Genome-wide analysis of genetic variation

Recently, it has used important "omics" techniques such as genomics, proteomics, host metabolomics, and oral microbiota metagenomics to well understand the progression of periodontitis [36]. Genome-wide association studies (GWAS) have been applied to detect genetic variations, from a large set of SNPs overall DNA, that are correlated with periodontitis [37, 38]. Many novel genes have been identified by GWAS studies for susceptibility of periodontitis, including NIN, NPY, and WNT5A in severe chronic type, NCR2 and EMR1 in moderate chronic [39], and GLT6D1 in aggressive type [40].

GWAS has provided new insights into periodontitis etiology at the genome level to answer how pathogenesis is affected by the identified susceptibility genes. Genome-wide genetic variation analysis includes total gene transcript, which referred to as transcriptomics. It has been carried on periodontal tissues [41, 42]. Proteomics and metabolomics have also been conducted on gingival crevicular fluids or saliva to study the influence of proteins and metabolites on immune mechanisms [43, 44]. It is remarkable that not only the genetic programming can be reflected by transcripts, proteins, and metabolites levels, but also disease progression and the results of response to environmental factors. Gene expression is regulated by chemical modification on DNA and its associated proteins (histones), which referred to epigenetics.

Now, it is accepted that heritable changes can be caused by the environment. In other words, it is known that neoplastic changes, normal differentiation, and changes caused by infections and inflammation are all results of epigenetic modifications.

Epigenetics is described as chemical changes in gene expression patterns, without changes in the DNA sequence. These modifications are consequences of environmental response, thereby remodeling the chromatin and selectively activating or inactivating genes, and determining their expression during development [45].

3. Epigenetic modifications

3.1 DNA methylation

Nucleosome is a repeating structure in which the chromatin is coordinated around and tightly packaged in the nucleus. It consists of an octamer of (H2A, H2B, H3, and H4) histones [46]. N-terminal tail of every histone and the C-terminal tail of histone H2A stick out of nucleosomal structure facilitating post-translational modifications. These epigenetic changes play a critical role in condensing and decondensing the DNA according to gene activity, regulating gene transcription in disease onset and progression, and in maintaining the integrity of chromosomes in all cell cycle phases [46]. The nucleosomes are fairly distributed over the chromosomes, and recently there are advanced techniques that can predict where their positions are accurately. Significantly, post-translational modifications occur in histones at defined positions and strongly correlate to DNA activities [4]. For instance, the addition of trimethyl at lysine 4 in histone H3 (H3K4) activates gene transcription, while trimethylation at H3K9 and H3K27 represses the transcription [4].

The most well-distinguished epigenetic modification is DNA methylation, which is an active process catalyzed by DNA methyltransferase (DNMT) enzymes. These enzymes add methyl group at the 5th carbon of cytosine in CpG dinucleotides known as CpG islands, which are CpG-rich areas of the DNA. They exist mostly in the

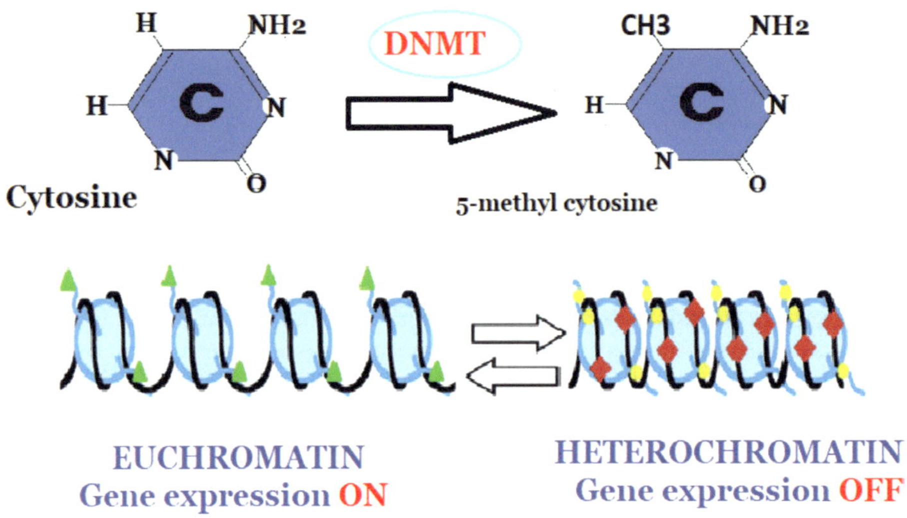

Figure 1.
represents DNA methylation on cytosine by DNA methyltransferase (DNMT) enzymes, leading to chromatin compaction (heterochromatin) and silencing gene expression.

promoter region of genes. Approximately, these CpG islands are noticed in 50% of human genes, and most of them are unmethylated in normal tissue [45].

Unmethylated CpGs are linked to transcriptionally active regions, whereas methylated DNA is promoted to interact with histone deacetylase enzymes (HDACs). HDAC enzyme removes acetyl groups of histones leading to compact the chromatin (heterochromatin) and then gene silencing because of prevention of transcription factor binding (**Figure 1**) [45]. Therefore, genes are not expressed. DNA methylation could regulate many cellular functions, including DNA repair and expression of inflammatory gene [47].

DNA methylation is maintained by DNMT1, and DNMT3a and DNMT3b mediate de novo methylation [48]. DNTM1 and HDAC activity are associated by making up a transcriptional repression complex. According to the role of DNMT1 and HDAC, their inhibitors could be therapeutic drugs in chronic inflammation [45].

3.2 Epigenetics of histone proteins

Epigenetic changes to the histones are caused by post-translational covalent modifications. Histone acetylation is catalyzed by histone acetyltransferase (HAT) enzymes which hold an acetyl group from acetyl-CoA to amino groups of lysine in histones. Covalent acetylation of histone leads to an open chromatin (euchromatin) which facilitates gene transcription by increasing transcription factor binding [49].

On the contrary, histone deacetylases (HDACs) remove acetyl groups from histones to form heterochromatin conformation which represses gene transcription [49]. In inflammatory, euchromatin activates genes of innate immune, whereas conformation of heterochromatin could suppress these genes. Hence, processes of the acetylation (by HAT) and deacetylation (by HDAC) must be matched to preserve immune homeostasis by the prevention of abnormal transcriptional activation or repression [49, 50].

Histone methylation is catalyzed by methyltransferase enzymes. Methylation of H3 histone is the most principal variation that includes H3 lysine 4 (H3K4), H3K9, H3K27,

H3K36, H3K79, and H4K20. H3K4me1 presents enhancer functions, and H3K27me3 is correlated with gene repression. These methylation processes may affect the disease by mediating regulation of cell cycle, DNA damage and development, and differentiation [51]. Histone methylation in aging tissue may lead to stem cell dysfunction. This may explain why chronic inflammations are popular in older people. Differential histone methylation could influence T cell inflammatory responses [52, 53].

For instance, in the presence of H3K27m3, interleukin-4 (IL4) and IL17 genes in Th1 cells and interferon-gamma (IFNG) gene in Th2 cells have been silenced. Histone methylation presents an important effect in controlling allogenic immune responses in graft-versus-host-disease (GVHD) [45].

Demethylating H3K27me3 at jumonji domain by JMJD3 histone demethylase regulates gene expression. Several studies have indicated the important roles of JMJD3 in numerous human diseases, such as infections, immune diseases, developmental diseases and cancer [54], and enhancing STAT6 gene expression upon IL-4 treatment [55].

H2A and B histones are changed by ubiquitination in cells and play an essential role in stem cell homeostasis by controlling gene pluripotency and differentiation, DNA repair, and X-chromosome deactivation [56].

Phosphorylation is another histone modification important in gene regulation. Histones are phosphorylated in cell cycle regulation in the physical state of chromatin maintaining. Researches presented that phosphorylation of histone H3 at Ser 10, 28, and Thr 11 activates transcription. Inflammation could activate tyrosine kinase, Janus kinase 2 (JAK2) which can directly phosphorylate Tyr 41 on H3 to stimulate specific genes transcription. That links histone phosphorylation to immune signaling [45].

3.3 RNA modifications

Among post-transcriptional modifications that regulate gene expression of an immune response, there are three mechanisms, RNA splicing, mRNA polyadenylation, and regulatory molecules, which include microRNA and long non-coding RNAs. The first mechanism is mRNA transcript modification when DNA is transcribed into mRNA. This process is called splicing, which removes non-coding sequences of mRNA (introns). Splicing patterns can be altered by bacterial products resulting in different protein isoforms [57].

After splicing, at the terminal end of the transcript, mRNA gains a sequence of adenosine bases called a poly(A)tail. This poly(A) tail length detects mRNA stability and the amount of mRNA transferred to the cytoplasm. It is also a way to maintain silenced mRNA within cell cytoplasm. In bacterial infection, cells can response rapidly by using silenced mRNA to induce gene expression without any need to retranscript DNA in the nucleus. This was also advocated as a mechanism to bind immune response to prevent chronic inflammatory inducing [57].

MicroRNA (miRNA) is a small non-coding molecule of RNA obtained from cleavage of longer RNA transcripts. It could regulate and fine-tune gene expression by a sequence-pairing homology to mRNA. When it binds to mRNA, it could repress the expression. Bacterial products and inflammatory cytokines can modify miRNA expression [57].

Recently, the long non-coding RNAs (lncRNAs) were discovered as another class of non-coding RNAs. lncRNAs involve in many biological roles. They bind to chromatin regulatory proteins, adjusting binding of these proteins to enhancer regions in the DNA, thereby regulating gene expression [57]. These RNAs function in the immune response involve host response regulation, including innate immunity since virus infection modifies lncRNAs expression. Chronic inflammations, such as periodontitis, have particular target tissues to destroy. Epigenetic patterns differ in each gene depending on the cell type, resulting in local and systemic gene expression [57].

This presents a site-specific change in the immune response to external stimuli, which may vary between patients and increase disease susceptibility. At last, we can say that studying immune genes and their susceptibility to epigenetic and genetic modification could define the vulnerability of periodontitis development.

4. Epigenetics in complex diseases

Continuously, there is new evidence showing the valuable role of epigenetic profiles in disease development and thus in diagnosis and treatment. GWAS have demonstrated that epigenetic alterations in tissues exposed to stress and extrinsic environmental factors give insight into cell response mechanism [58]. These studies also provide information about cell dealing with these alterations, what the risk factors involved, and whether they can be treated, or lead to cell apoptosis. GWAS has detected association between genetic and epigenetics modification and the susceptibility and progression of the disease [58]. Extensive analysis has been performed to determine gene expression profiles and/or loci modified epigenetically to identify which are associated with a specific disease [59]. Epigenetic marks and clinical outcomes combination enhances the vision about the prediction of the disease and therapeutic target determination. And yet it is more a perception than a reality in medicine nowadays.

5. Epigenetics in environmental response

Each tissue including embryonic stem cells has a specific epigenetic pattern, and upon processes of development and regeneration this pattern modifies. Epigenetic pattern modifications are influenced by external factors that involve in differentiation, like hormones [60]. So we can say that these patterns are reflection of the tissue activity in defined time and its gene expression profile.

Experiments on induced pluripotent stem cells have proved that treatment could generate a specific epigenetic profile. Microbiota could trigger an immune response by excreting signals that are able to change that profile. In gingival tissues, microbial signals combined with external risk factors from food intake and smoking could make a similar effect on epigenetic profile [61].

6. Epigenetics in periodontitis

Epigenetics is a relatively fresh thought in periodontitis studies. This concept could reveal the lost relationship between disease, genetics, and environment. It is clear that periodontitis is most common in the elderly, but recently researches have presented that some types of this disease like gingivitis, may develop at any age [62].

Each tissue can have a special epigenetic pattern, and alterations depend on regenerative and progression processes. For instance, there is certain indication that the epigenetic profile of embryonic stem cells changes upon differentiation [63]. Continuously, the oral mucosa is exposed to pathogens and microflora. Gingival cells must distinguish both of them and prompt inflammatory responses only to pathogens. It is already well proved that periodontium inflammation is induced by the microbial biofilm [62]. Its continuous fluster causes to constant apoptosis, thereby tissue regeneration process that may enforce unique epigenetic alterations resulting in a different phenotype. External environmental factors, growth factors, and hormones that regulate differentiation may lead to these epigenetic modifications [64].

Oral hygiene is certainly a key factor to healthy gingiva and decreases the inflammatory condition. Lifestyle of smoking, malnutrition, lack of physical activity, and drug use heavily affect the epigenetic profile leading to many diseases, including periodontal disease. Chronic periodontitis needs elevated production of gingiva cells such as epithelial cells, fibroblasts, and osteoblasts to compensate for cell death. Cell proliferating imperfection may cause abnormal response, which in turn leads to a motley phenotype [65].

In fact, periodontal disease is identified by site susceptibility with certain areas showing the majority of the disease and others being healthy. Epigenetic modifications could happen at specific regions or affect most of the periodontium. Accumulation of site plaque may explain site prediction, but still after treatment and with high hygiene these sites' susceptibility remains, and epigenetics explain their inflammatory responsiveness alteration [45].

It has been pointed out that the inflammatory response in periodontitis is similar to other inflammatory diseases, where transcription factors upregulation and signal transducer and activator of transcription (STAT), and chromatin changes occur that might induce epigenetic modifications [66].

6.1 DNA methylation in periodontal disease

In periodontitis, as we already mentioned that the epigenome differs between inflamed and unflamed periodontal tissues in the same person. In addition, different methylation profiles correlated with regulating apoptosis, cell differentiation, lipopolysaccharide-mediated signaling, and oncogenesis pathways were presented in inflamed sites compared to healthy ones.

Many studies have searched for methylation of cytokine genes in periodontitis. Analysis of the IL-8 promoter suggests a tissue-specific profile in DNA methylation. In epithelial cells, the methylation frequency of IL-8 was altered in patients when compared with controls, but no difference was noticed in gingival cells or blood leukocytes. It was found that IL-6 promoter partially methylated in both controls and patients, with higher level of IL-6 expression in periodontitis subjects [67]. Increased IL-6 serum level in chronic periodontitis patients was correlated with hypomethylation of the −74 bp CpG site in the IL-6 promoter. This shows that single CpG site methylation may affect the production of cytokines and thus disease [68].

Studies have reported a lower methylation level of CpG sites in IFN-γ promoter in periodontitis compared to healthy tissues. This was associated with rising IFN-γ transcription [68]. The increase was independent of promoter methylation. Regarding the IL-10 gene, three CpG islands near to the promoter around the −1087 polymorphism were methylated in peripheral blood cells and gingival tissues. B cells treatment with 5-aza-deoxycytidine (5-aza), the inhibitor of DNA methylation, increased IL-10 mRNA whatever the genotype of the −1087 SNP [69].

Hypermethylation of two CpG islands in the TNF-α promoter was defined in chronic periodontitis. Treatment of ThP1 cells with the 5-aza regulated TNF-α transcription and raised TNF-α expression [57].

Not only cytokine methylation level has been investigated in periodontitis, but also some other genes linked to inflammation. The pattern of DNA methylation in the toll-like receptor-2 (TLR2) and TLR4 genes was estimated in gingival tissues. Their results showed major unmethylation of the TLR4 gene promoter, but the TLR2 gene promoter was found as a mosaic of methylated and unmethylated DNA in the majority of samples. Hypermethylation and a subsequent reduced expression of TLR2 in periodontitis tissues was reported. A positive association was found between periodontal probing depth and TLR2 methylation [70].

E-Cadherin and COX-2 genes methylation status was studied in breast cancer and chronic periodontitis patients and compared hypermethylation between both diseases and healthy people [71]. The thought that cancer and chronic inflammation may have an identical epigenetic profile was proved. This was shown that DNA methylation may be a connection between cancer and inflammation.

Zhang et al. study illustrates a mechanism on how gene expression may be affected by DNA methylation of a gene promoter. It has shown that inflammation causes hypermethylation of PTGS2 promoter which correlated with reduced levels of its gene transcription [72]. Interestingly, a highly methylated CpG island was found close to the binding site of transcription factor, suggesting that methylation status may prevent the binding of NFκB [72]. This is in accordance with other studies on methylation of cytokine promoters in which the CpG islands analyzed were in close proximity to transcription factors NFκB and Sp1 binding sites [73]. NFκB and Sp1 regulate gene expression of the immune response. They are activated by bacteria binding to TLRs and the subsequent activation of mitogen-activated protein kinase (MAPK) pathways. Binding of Sp1 and NFκB to adjacent sites influenced nucleosomes repositioning upstream and downstream of the factors, thereby inducing gene transcription. It has been proved that extracellular signal transduction pathways regulate methylation enzymes, such as the MAPK ERK kinase pathway [57].

Abnormal DNA methylation in tissues has been caused by inflammation. This mechanism has been a correlation between periodontitis and changes in methylation level in cancer. In infected tissues, eosinophils and neutrophils create materials that can halogenate cytosine. Halogenated cytosine and methylated DNA cannot be differentiated by DNMT1 enzyme, thereby de novo methylation increases in cells of inflamed tissues [74].

6.2 Histone modifications and periodontitis

Gene expression is regulated by post-translational histone alterations, such as acetylation/deacetylation, methylation, and phosphorylation, that have an epigenetic role in chromatin organization. Studies have presented a relationship between histone acetylation and cardiovascular diseases. Regarding inflammation, several genes of pro-inflammatory cytokines are managed by interacting with some transcription factors, such as NF-kB, SP1, and AP-1. As these factors are activated, they bind to particular response elements on the gene promoter and interact with co-activators with HAT activity to control gene transcriptional activity [75].

In inflammation, it has been shown that lysine residues acetylation on histone H4 increases gene expression of pro-inflammatory cytokines such as IL-1B and TNF. An experiment has applied by using trichostatin A (TSA) in airway epithelial cells which is able to inhibit HDACs. It has resulted in increased inflammatory signals, which confirms HDACs role in inflammatory gene repression [76].

Although very few observations, histone modifications are also implicated in periodontitis. Maintenance of histone acetylation of genes correlated to osteoclastogenesis has been found to be crucial to prevent bone loss in periodontitis. Treatment with HDACs inhibitor has improved bone levels [77].

When stimulated with *P. gingivalis* and *F. nucleatum*, gingival epithelial cells presented differential expression of HDAC1, HDAC2, DNMT1 genes, and H3 Lys 4 methylation. Studies have suggested that *P. gingivalis* and epigenetics interact together to regulate immune response, and a correlation between LPS stimulation and histone alteration has been found [78].

7. Therapeutic approach and future perspectives

Researches have investigated patient care benefit in relation to current therapeutics in inflammations. Indeed, clinicians could incorporate some of the advances in epigenetics and anti-inflammatory management procedures to improve diagnosis and treatment of periodontal diseases. Epigenetic alterations previously discussed could benefit in better diagnosis, and some of them are worth highlighted.

Epigenetic processes evolutionarily give an equilibrium in gene regulation. However, abnormal alterations of epigenetics may cause major problems in inflammations. The studies governing epigenetic modifications may answer to periodontitis initiation and progression. For example, methylation levels in genes and miRNA targeting may be utilized as possible biomarkers for the periodontitis severity. Clinicians may use, in addition to their diagnostic methods, identifying SNPs related with high disease susceptibility. The etiological similarities between periodontitis and other immune diseases have made it possible to develop potential new therapeutic approaches [79].

Actually, many studies aim to discover new targeted drugs regarding the exact inflammatory and genetic factors of periodontitis progression. Inhibitors of histone deacetylase (HDACs) and DNA methyltransferase (DNMTs) could affect periodontal therapy positively [79]. The main warning is that currently, the epigenetic reprogramming drugs are not targeted and site-specific, even so, 5-Aza-2′-deoxycytidine (decitabine) as a demethylation drug could shift methylated genes in the inflammatory system [80].

More experiments are necessary to confirm targeting drugs at a goal loci. Suberoylanilide hydroxamic acid (SAHA), approved HDAC inhibitor, represses class 1 and 2 of HDACs. SAHA increases histone acetylation, which unwinds the chromatin and induces gene expression. Histone methyltransferase inhibitor (HMTase) inhibits histone methyltransferase EZH2 and activates tumor suppressor gene expression including specific inflammatory genes [81].

Bromodomain and extraterminal domain (BET) proteins are a group of epigenetic regulatory proteins that can read acetylated histone tails and contribute to gene transcription regulation. Recently, the BET inhibitor JQ1 was suggested to be a potential treatment model for periodontitis. It represses both an immune response and alveolar bone loss in periodontitis. Experiments have demonstrated that JQ1 decreases BET protein binding to the NFκB promoters, leading to reduce NFκB transcription [82].

Aspirin has a negative effect on allergic inflammation by regulating DNMT1 expression. Aspirin could prevent antigen from modifying HDAC3 and DNMT1 expression [83].

8. Stem cells and periodontitis

Recently, stem cells have been considered as a new tissue-engineering treatment approach. Various studies have demonstrated that these cells have regenerative and immunomodulatory properties make them applicable in inflammation treatment. The immunomodulatory properties are due to secretion of extracellular vesicles (EVs) that are membrane-bound compounds. EVs have the ability to transport DNA, peptides, and lipids that may influence target cell activity and non-coding RNA leading to gene expression modifications. EVs could offer a prolong therapy free of cells, to avoid immunogenicity reduction and tumorigenesis risk. Also, they play as a carrier of therapeutics [84].

Mesenchymal stem cells (MSCs) have several tissue sources, such as umbilical cord, bone marrow, or adipose tissue [85]. Furthermore, many stem cell subtypes have been isolated from gingival and ligament tissues called dental mesenchymal stem cells (DMSCs) [86]. DMSCs are pluripotent have the ability to renew and differentiate into numerous cell types. They could alter activity of immune-related cells depending on many factors secreted by immune cells [87]. Because of pathogens of periodontitis and inflammatory response, stem cell effects and their osteogenic differentiation are suppressed.

OCN and Runx2 genes involved in osteogenic have reduced expression in inflammatory tissues. Abnormal osteogenic differentiation in ligament stem cells is influenced by epigenetic alterations. Hypermethylation of bone development genes reduces their expression [88].

8.1 Stem cells and periodontal tissue regeneration

Alveolar bone resorption, a characteristic of periodontitis, needs regenerative therapy. It is caused by imbalance of bone homeostasis which upgrade osteoclastogenesis. Nuclear factor kappa light-chain enhancer of activated B cells (NFκB) has involved in this process. Stem cells could be a great pathway for regeneration and bone loss repression.

Experiments have presented that biomarks expressed by PDLSCs are correlated with osteoblasts and cementoblasts. Injection of MSCs derived from gingiva has reduced bone resorption in mice after 1 month [89]. Similarly, it is shown that BM-MSCs therapy could reduce osteoclastogenesis by repression of mRNA expression of the receptor activator of NFκB (RANKL) [90].

Another study demonstrated that treatment with MSCs in fibroin/chitosan hydrogel in rats induced alveolar bone gain [91]. Furthermore, new tissue formation can be promoted by mediators secreted from MSCs such as cytokines and growth factor, and EVs. Studies have proved that MSC-EVs associated with increased bone volume [92]. Numerous researches have proved the critical role of stem cells and their products in bone homeostasis modulation. For example, PDLSCs and GMSCs secrete exosomes that could disturb Wnt pathway expression, leading to induce osteogenic differentiation [93, 94].

Additionally, modulation of mesenchymal stem cells could promote EVs production with overexpressed materials. In periodontal experiment on mice, exosomes from bone marrow MSCs charged with miR-26a have the ability to induce differentiation of osteogenic and improve new bone formation [95].

Interestingly, studies have compared the potential role in osteogenic between PDLSCs, dental follicle progenitor cells, and dental pulp stem cells. Genes related to osteogenic were upregulated, and their osteogenic ability was higher [96].

Furthermore, it has presented that PDLSCs could improve osteogenic differentiation in other cells [84]. Additionally, other stem cell types could affect the infected microenvironment, like bone marrow stem cells that cause repression of T lymphocyte proliferation using IFN-γ. The transplantation of stimulated BMSCs repressed cytokine production, inflammatory tissue destruction, and new tissue formation [84]. The important role of stem cells is due to their proliferation capacity and ability to migrate and differentiate, and immunosuppressive properties in the inflamed microenvironment [97].

9. Conclusions

Although many questions remain, epigenetic modifications are important targets for developing new drugs of periodontitis. Experimental periodontitis *in vivo* can provide insights into understanding bacterial-induced disease-specific epigenetic changes in histone changes and/or DNA methylation that may indicate new therapeutic targets.

MSCs and their EVs have induced bone loss repression. EVs secreted from healthy stem cells are able to improve cell reformation properties in inflamed tissues. This promising role could be benefit in clinical application of periodontal therapy controlling the inflammation through non-surgical and surgical treatments. However, the therapeutic success needs many factors that include the microenvironment, stem cell sources, the experimental design, and the procedures and protocol of isolation and transplantation. Also, it should clarify the inclusion and exclusion criteria.

Acronyms and abbreviations

MSCs	Mesenchymal stem cells
SNP	Single nucleotide polymorphism
DEFB	Defensins
TLR-2	Toll-like receptor-2
FCGR2A	Fc-γ receptor
IL-1	Interleukin-1
TNFA	Tumor necrosis factor alpha
MMP	Matrix metalloproteinase
COX-2	cyclo-oxygenase-2
GWAS	Genome-wide association studies
DNMT	DNA methyltransferase
HDACs	Histone deacetylases
HATs	Histone acetyltransferases
IFNG	Interferon gamma
GVHD	Graft-versus-host-disease
JAK2	Janus kinase 2
miRNAs	microRNAs
lncRNAs	Long non-coding RNAs
STAT	Signal transducer and activator of transcription
LPS	Lipopolysaccharide
5-aza	5-aza-deoxycytidine
MAPK	Mitogen-activated protein kinase

EVs	Extracellular vesicles
DMSCs	Dental mesenchymal stem cells
NFκB	Nuclear factor kappa light-chain enhancer of activated B cells
RANKL	Receptor activator of NFκB

Author details

Faten Kafa
Damascus University, Damascus, Syrian Arab Republic

*Address all correspondence to: faten.kafa@damascusuniversity.edu.sy

References

[1] Stabholz A, Soskolne WA, Shapira LJP. Genetic and environmental risk factors for chronic periodontitis and aggressive periodontitis. Periodontology 2000. 2010;**53**(1):138-153

[2] Wiebe CB, Putnins EE. The periodontal disease classification system of the American Academy of periodontology-an update. Journal of the Canadian Dental Association. 2000;**66**(11):594-599

[3] Armitage GC. Development of a classification system for periodontal diseases and conditions. Annals of Periodontology. 2000;**79**(6):31-35

[4] Lindroth AM, Park YJ. Epigenetic biomarkers: A step forward for understanding periodontitis. Journal of Periodontal & Implant Science. 2013;**43**(3):111-120

[5] Jilani M et al. Association between vitamin D receptor gene polymorphisms and chronic periodontitis among Libyans. Libyan Journal of Medicine. 2015;**10**:1

[6] Kafa F, Abou Sulaiman A, Haddad S. Association of matrix metalloproteinase-8 gene promoter polymorphisms with type II diabetes mellitus in Syrian population. Human Gene. 2022;**33**:201061

[7] Genco RJ, Van Dyke TE. Reducing the risk of CVD in patients with periodontitis. Nature Reviews Cardiology. 2010;**7**(9):479-480

[8] Nibali L et al. Association between metabolic syndrome and periodontitis: A systematic review and meta-analysis. The Journal of Clinical Endocrinology & Metabolism. 2013;**98**(3):913-920

[9] Awano S et al. Oral health and mortality risk from pneumonia in the elderly. Journal of Dental Research. 2008;**87**(4):334-339

[10] Van Dyke TE, Dave S. Risk factors for periodontitis. Journal of the International Academy of Periodontology. 2005;**7**(1):3

[11] Kafa F, Abou Sulaiman A, Haddad S. Association between vitamin D receptor FOKI polymorphism and chronic periodontitis in Syrian population. International Journal of Pharmaceutical Sciences and Research. 2019;**10**(3):1336-1341

[12] Brodzikowska A, Górski B. Polymorphisms in genes involved in inflammation and periodontitis: A narrative review. Biomolecules. 2022;**12**(4):552

[13] Heidari Z, Moudi B, Mahmoudzadeh-Sagheb H. Immunomodulatory factors gene polymorphisms in chronic periodontitis: An overview. BMC Oral Health. 2019;**19**(1):1-15

[14] Shao J et al. DEFB1 rs11362 polymorphism and risk of chronic periodontitis: A meta-analysis of unadjusted and adjusted data. Frontiers in Genetics. 2019;**10**:179

[15] Kozak M et al. Cytokines and their genetic polymorphisms related to periodontal disease. Journal of Clinical Medicine. 2020;**9**(12):4045

[16] Mehlotra RK et al. Associations of toll-like receptor and β-defensin polymorphisms with measures of periodontal disease (PD) in HIV+ North American adults: An exploratory study. PLoS One. 2016;**11**(10):e0164075

[17] Vahabi S et al. Investigating the association between rs4986790 polymorphism of TLR4 gene and chronic periodontitis in an Iranian population: TLR4 gene polymorphism and chronic periodontitis. Journal of Dental School. 2022;**40**(4):159-165

[18] Chai L et al. SNPs of fc-gamma receptor genes and chronic periodontitis. Journal of Dental Research. 2010;**89**(7):705-710

[19] Shibani K, Shhab R, Khattab R. Analysis of IL-1α (– 889) and IL-1B (+ 3953) gene polymorphism in Syrian patients with aggressive periodontitis: A pilot study. ISRN Dentistry. 2011;**2011**:1-5

[20] Brodzikowska A, Górski B, Bogusławska-Kapała A. Association between IL-1 gene polymorphisms and stage III grade B periodontitis in polish population. International Journal of Environmental Research and Public Health. 2022;**19**(22):14687

[21] Brodzikowska A, Górska R, Kowalski J. Interleukin-1 genotype in periodontitis. Archivum Immunologiae et Therapiae Experimentalis. 2019;**67**:367-373

[22] Cirelli T et al. Genetic polymorphisms in the interleukins IL1B, IL4, and IL6 are associated with concomitant periodontitis and type 2 diabetes mellitus in Brazilian patients. Journal of Periodontal Research. 2020;**55**(6):918-930

[23] dos Santos EC et al. Study of TNF-α, IFN-γ, TGF-β, IL-6, and IL-10 gene polymorphism in individuals from the leprosy endemic area in the Brazilian Amazon. Meta Gene. 2020;**25**:100740

[24] Mehar R et al. Interleukin-6 gene-174G> C promoter polymorphism reduces the risk of periodontitis in Brazilian populations: A meta-analysis. Journal of Oral Biosciences. 2021;**63**(4):388-393

[25] Chrysanthakopoulos N. The role of inflammatory cytokines and interleukin-6 expression gene polymorphism in chronic periodontitis: Review of the literature. Journal of Clinical Case Reports and Medical Research. 2020;**1**:4

[26] Stolf CS et al. IL10 promoter rs6667202 polymorphism is functional in health but not in grade c periodontitis patients: A pilot study. Journal of Periodontal Research. 2022;**57**(1):85-93

[27] Shan C et al. Association of polymorphism in IL-18 gene with periodontitis in Uyghur adults in Xinjiang and evidence from six case-control studies with a comprehensive analysis. A Journal of Molecular and Cellular Immunology. 2022;**51**(3):511-530

[28] Mazurek-Mochol M et al. IL-18 gene rs187238 and rs1946518 polymorphisms and expression in gingival tissue in patients with periodontitis. Biomedicine. 2022;**10**(10):2367

[29] Du F, Liu Z, Qing S. Effect of vitamin D receptor gene polymorphisms on the risk of chronic and aggressive periodontitis: A systematic review and meta-analysis of the Chinese population. Archives of Oral Biology. 2022;**144**:105566

[30] Shi LX et al. Association between TNF-α G-308A (rs1800629) polymorphism and susceptibility to chronic periodontitis and type 2 diabetes mellitus: A meta-analysis. Journal of Periodontal Research. 2021;**56**(2):226-235

[31] Li Y et al. TNF-α polymorphisms might influence predisposition to periodontitis: A meta-analysis. Microbial Pathogenesis. 2020;**143**:104113

[32] Kafa F, Abou Sulaiman A, Haddad S. Association of tumor necrosis factor-α gene promoter polymorphisms with periodontitis in type II diabetic Syrian population. International Journal of Dentistry and Oral Science. 2021;**8**(11):5064-5069

[33] Alotaibi DH et al. The association of matrix metalloproteinase gene polymorphisms and periodontitis: An overview. Journal of Pharmacy and Bioallied Sciences. 2020;**12**(Suppl. 1): S37-S42

[34] Saremi L et al. Evaluation of matrix metalloproteinase-1,-2,-3,-7, and-13 gene polymorphisms in patients with chronic periodontitis and healthy controls. Clinical Oral Investigations. 2023;**27**(12):7417-7423

[35] Gholami M et al. Association of periodontitis and aging-related diseases: A review of mechanistic studies. Journal of Research in Dental and Maxillofacial Sciences. 2023;**8**(1):62-70

[36] Grant MM. What do'omic technologies have to offer periodontal clinical practice in the future? Journal of Periodontal Research. 2012;**47**(1):2-14

[37] Petty LE et al. Genome-wide association study identifies novel risk loci for apical periodontitis. Journal of Endodontics. 2023;**49**(10): 1276-1288

[38] de Coo A et al. Genome-wide association study of stage III/IV grade C periodontitis (former aggressive periodontitis) in a Spanish population. Journal of Clinical Periodontology. 2021;**48**(7):896-906

[39] Divaris K et al. Exploring the genetic basis of chronic periodontitis: A genome-wide association study. Human Molecular Genetics. 2013;**22**(11):2312-2324

[40] Schaefer AS et al. A genome-wide association study identifies GLT6D1 as a susceptibility locus for periodontitis. Human Molecular Genetics. 2010;**19**(3):553-562

[41] Lundmark A et al. Gene expression profiling of periodontitis-affected gingival tissue by spatial transcriptomics. Scientific Reports. 2018;**8**(1):9370

[42] Kebschull M et al. Gingival tissue transcriptomes identify distinct periodontitis phenotypes. Journal of Dental Research. 2014;**93**(5):459-468

[43] Bonne NJ, Wong DTW. Salivary biomarker development using genomic, proteomic and metabolomic approaches. Genome Medicine. 2012;**4**(10):1-12

[44] Baima G et al. Metabolomics of gingival crevicular fluid to identify biomarkers for periodontitis: A systematic review with meta-analysis. Journal of Periodontal Research. 2021;**56**(4):633-645

[45] Benakanakere MR et al. Epigenetics, inflammation, and periodontal disease. Current Oral Health Reports. 2019;**6**:37-46

[46] Morrison O, Thakur J. Molecular complexes at euchromatin, heterochromatin and centromeric chromatin. International Journal of Molecular Sciences. 2021;**22**(13):6922

[47] Gomez RS, Dutra WO, Moreira PR. Epigenetics and periodontal disease: Future perspectives. Inflammation Research. 2009;**58**:625-629

[48] Seaborne RAE. The role of DNA methylation in the regulation of skeletal muscle atrophy, hypertrophy and epigenetic 'Memory' [ProQuest dissertation & theses]. United Kingdom: Liverpool John Moores University; 2018

[49] Jiang N et al. Acetylation in pathogenesis: Revealing emerging mechanisms and therapeutic prospects. Biomedicine & Pharmacotherapy. 2023;**167**:115519

[50] Smale ST, Tarakhovsky A, Natoli G. Chromatin contributions to the regulation of innate immunity. Annual Review of Immunology. 2014;**32**:489-511

[51] Huang Y et al. Global mapping of H3K4me3 and H3K27me3 reveals chromatin state-based regulation of human monocyte-derived dendritic cells in different environments. Genes and Immunity. 2012;**13**(4):311-320

[52] Francis M et al. Histone methylation: Achilles heel and powerful mediator of periodontal homeostasis. Journal of Dental Research. 2020;**99**(12):1332-1340

[53] Liaw A et al. The relevance of DNA methylation and histone modification in periodontitis: A scoping review. Cells. 2022;**11**(20):3211

[54] Jin Y et al. Histone demethylase JMJD3 downregulation protects against aberrant force-induced osteoarthritis through epigenetic control of NR4A1. International Journal of Oral Science. 2022;**14**(1):34

[55] De Santa F et al. The histone H3 lysine-27 demethylase Jmjd3 links inflammation to inhibition of polycomb-mediated gene silencing. Cell Journal. 2007;**130**(6):1083-1094

[56] Hosseini A, Minucci S. Alterations of histone modifications in cancer. In: Epigenetics in Human Disease. 2nd ed. Translational Epigenetics Series. Vol. 6. ScienceDirect; 2018. pp. 141-217

[57] Larsson L, Castilho RM, Giannobile WV. Epigenetics and its role in periodontal diseases: A state-of-the-art review. Journal of Periodontology. 2015;**86**(4):556-568

[58] Lopez-Lopez E. Genetics and epigenetics in complex diseases. International Journal of Molecular Sciences. 2023;**24**(9):8186

[59] Trejo Banos D et al. Bayesian reassessment of the epigenetic architecture of complex traits. Nature Communications. 2020;**11**(1):2865

[60] Lardon R, Geelen DJP. Natural variation in plant pluripotency and regeneration. Plants. 2020;**9**(10):1261

[61] Hochedlinger K, Jaenisch R. Induced pluripotency and epigenetic reprogramming. Cold Spring Harbor Perspectives in Biology. 2015;**7**(12):a019448

[62] Gasner NS, Schure RS. Periodontal disease. In: StatPearls. NCBI Bookshelf; 2023

[63] Trapp A, Kerepesi C, Gladyshev VN. Profiling epigenetic age in single cells. Nature Aging. 2021;**1**(12):1189-1201

[64] Cortessis VK et al. Environmental epigenetics: Prospects for studying epigenetic mediation of exposure–response relationships. Human Genetics. 2012;**131**:1565-1589

[65] Lod S et al. The influence of epigenetics in relation to oral health. International Journal of Dental Hygiene. 2014;**12**(1):48-54

[66] Larsson L. Current concepts of epigenetics and its role in periodontitis. Current Oral Health Reports. 2017;**4**:286-293

[67] Huang J, Wang Y, Zhou Y. METTL3 and METTL14 regulate IL-6

expression via RNA m6A modification of zinc transporter SLC39A9 and DNA methylation of IL-6 in periodontal ligament cells. Biochimica et Biophysica Acta (BBA)-Molecular Cell Research. 2024;**1871**(1):119605

[68] Jiang Y et al. DNA methylation alterations and their potential influence on macrophage in periodontitis. Oral Diseases. 2022;**28**(2):249-263

[69] Yang W, Thompson B, Kwa FAA. Molecular approaches for the treatment and prevention of Friedreich's ataxia. Drug Discovery Today. 2022;**27**(3):866-880

[70] Bordagaray MJ et al. CpG single-site methylation regulates TLR2 expression in proinflammatory PBMCs from apical periodontitis individuals. Frontiers in Immunology. 2022;**13**:861665

[71] Khouly I et al. The role of epigenetics in periodontal and systemic diseases and smoking: A systematic review. Applied Sciences. 2021;**11**(11):5269

[72] Zhang S et al. Alteration of PTGS2 promoter methylation in chronic periodontitis. Journal of Dental Research. 2010;**89**(2):133-137

[73] Zhang S et al. Epigenetic regulation of TNFA expression in periodontal disease. Journal of Periodontology. 2013;**84**(11):1606-1616

[74] Baljinnyam T et al. Chemical and enzymatic modifications of 5-methylcytosine at the intersection of DNA damage, repair, and epigenetic reprogramming. PLoS One. 2022;**17**(8):e0273509

[75] Hinson AN et al. Treponema denticola induces in-terleukin-36γ expression in human oral gingival keratinocytes via the parallel activation of NF-kB and mitogen-activated protein kinase pathways. Infection and Immunity. 2022;**90**(10):e00247-22

[76] Jurdziński KT, Potempa J, Grabiec AM. Epigenetic regulation of inflammation in periodontitis: Cellular mechanisms and therapeutic potential. Clinical Epigenetics. 2020;**12**(1):1-18

[77] Zhao Q et al. Effect of the histone deacetylases inhibitors on the differentiation of stem cells in bone damage repairing and regeneration. Current Stem Cell Research & Therapy. 2020;**15**(1):24-31

[78] Yin L, Chung W. Epigenetic regulation of human-defensin 2 and CC chemokine ligand 20 expression in gingival epithelial cells in response to oral bacteria. Mucosal Immunology. 2011;**4**(4):409-419

[79] Laberge S et al. The Potential Role of Epigenetic Modifications on Different Facets in the Periodontal Pathogenesis. 2023;**14**(6):1202

[80] Tanaka U et al. Decitabine inhibits bone resorption in periodontitis by upregulating anti-inflammatory cytokines and suppressing osteoclastogenesis. Biomedicine. 2021;**9**(2):199

[81] Sulistyowati I. Histone deacetylase inhibitor induces the odontogenic differentiation in human dental pulp cells: Comparison of trichostatin a (TSA) and suberoylanilide hydroxamic acid (SAHA). In: Oral Biology and Oral Pathology Commons. Chulalongkorn University Theses and Dissertations (Chula Etd); 2020

[82] Sun M et al. Selective BET inhibitor RVX-208 ameliorates periodontal inflammation and bone loss. Journal of Clinical Periodontology. 2023;**50**(12):1658-1669

[83] Shi Y et al. Aspirin loaded extracellular vesicles inhibit inflammation of macrophages via switching metabolic phenotype in periodontitis. Biochemical and Biophysical Research Communications. 2023;**667**:25-33

[84] Ustianowska K et al. The genetic aspects of periodontitis pathogenesis and the regenerative properties of stem cells. Cells. 2024;**13**(2):117

[85] Hendijani F. Explant culture: An advantageous method for isolation of mesenchymal stem cells from human tissues. Cell Proliferation. 2017;**50**(2):e12334

[86] Gan L et al. Dental tissue-derived human mesenchymal stem cells and their potential in therapeutic application. Stem Cells International. 2020;**2020**:1-17

[87] Wang L et al. Characterization of stem cells from alveolar periodontal ligament. Tissue Engineering Part A. 2011;**17**(7-8):1015-1026

[88] Adithya SP, Balagangadharan K, Selvamurugan N. Epigenetic modifications of histones during osteoblast differentiation. Biochimica et Biophysica Acta (BBA)-Gene Regulatory Mechanisms. 2022;**1865**(1):194780

[89] Sun W et al. The treatment of systematically transplanted gingival mesenchymal stem cells in periodontitis in mice. Experimental and Therapeutic Medicine. 2019;**17**(3):2199-2205

[90] Lu L et al. The therapeutic role of bone marrow stem cell local injection in rat experimental periodontitis. Journal of Oral Rehabilitation. 2020;**47**:73-82

[91] Balaban YE et al. Local application of gingiva-derived mesenchymal stem cells on experimental periodontitis in rats. Journal of Periodontology. 2024;**95**:456-468

[92] Zhou H et al. Mesenchymal stem cell-derived extracellular vesicles for treatment of bone loss within periodontitis in pre-clinical animal models: A meta-analysis. BMC Oral Health. 2023;**23**(1):701

[93] Nakao Y et al. Exosomes from TNF-α-treated human gingiva-derived MSCs enhance M2 macrophage polarization and inhibit periodontal bone loss. Acta Biomaterialia. 2021;**122**:306-324

[94] Lei F et al. Treatment of inflammatory bone loss in periodontitis by stem cell-derived exosomes. Acta Biomaterialia. 2022;**141**:333-343

[95] Lai S et al. Bone marrow mesenchymal stem cell-derived exosomes loaded with miR-26a through the novel immunomodulatory peptide DP7-C can promote osteogenesis. Biotechnology Letters. 2023;**45**(7):905-919

[96] Ai T et al. DNA methylation profile is associated with the osteogenic potential of three distinct human odontogenic stem cells. Signal Transduction and Targeted Therapy. 2018;**3**(1):1

[97] Bindal P et al. Immune responses of human dental pulp stem cells in lipopolysaccharide-induced microenvironment. Cell Biology International. 2018;**42**(7):832-840

Section 2

Advanced Diagnostic Techniques

Chapter 3

Benefits of Three-Dimensional Printing in Periodontal Therapy

Pitu Wulandari

Abstract

Periodontal disease is one of the most common dental and oral diseases suffered by people in the world, especially in Indonesia. The prevalence of this disease increases from year to year. The most important thing to prevent further destruction due to this disease is a correct and accurate diagnosis and treatment plan, one of which is using 3D (three-dimensional) printing in periodontal treatment. Three-dimensional printing is a process of building 3D objects by adding additional approaches. Using 3D printing, periodontal care procedures such as creating study models, scaffolds, preservation sockets, bone augmentation, and implant implantation can be completed.

Keywords: periodontal diseases, periodontal therapy, three-dimensional, printing, scaffolds

1. Introduction

Dentistry technology has developed rapidly. One of the newest technological innovations in dentistry is the use of three-dimensional (3D) printing [1]. 3D printing is considered a *disruptive technology* that has the power to change the way products are produced. Recently, 3D printing has become a subject of great interest in dentistry [2]. 3D printing allows small quantities of customized items to be produced at relatively low cost. While currently 3D printing is used primarily for prototyping and mock-ups, some promising applications exist in creating replacement parts, scaffolds, dental crowns, and artificial limbs, such as in manufacturing bridges [3].

The term 3D printing is generally used to describe a manufacturing approach that builds an object one layer at a time, adding multiple layers to the shape of an object. This process is more accurately described as additive manufacturing and is also referred to as rapid prototyping [2]. Technology is slowly continuing to make its way into the field of dentistry. Researchers continue to strive to integrate technology into the field of dentistry. Of all the latest technological innovations in dentistry, the most discussed innovation currently is three-dimensional (3D) bioprinting [4].

2. 3D printing

The first 3D object was printed by Charles Hull in 1983 using Stereolithography. Although Francois Duret introduced digital dentistry in the 1970s, it was not readily accepted and took time to be integrated into current dental practice. Hull later founded 3D Systems, which produces the premier 3D printer "Stereolithography Apparatus". In 1988, 3D Systems launched the SLA-250, the first commercially viable 3D printer [5, 6].

3D printing allows operators to produce objects with more complex designs and shapes using fewer materials than traditional manufacturing methods [7]. 3D printers work similarly to conventional laser or inkjet printers, rather than using colorful inks. 3D printers use a powdered or liquid resin that is slowly created from an image layer by layer. All 3D printers use 3D CAD (Computer-Aided Design) software that measures thousands of cross-sections of each product to determine exactly how each layer should be constructed. The 3D machine dispenses thin layers of liquid resin and uses computer-controlled ultraviolet lasers to harden each layer in a specified cross-sectional pattern. Excess soft resin is removed through a chemical bath at the end of the process [3]. 3D printing technology allows doctors to individually customize the production of body parts for the patient they are treating [7].

3. 3D printing technology

There are three main steps in carrying out the 3D printing process: the first step starts with data acquisition, namely obtaining a 3D object file. In the fabrication process using additive manufacturing technology, initially, 3D images are taken with the help of dental cone beam computer tomography or with medical magnetic resonance imaging, obtaining models from CBCT (Cone Beam Computed Tomography), MRI (Magnetic Resonance Imaging), or CT (Computed Tomography) [6]. Computed Tomography is then transferred to software for designing with the help of a computer, the second step is to create the data obtained with the help of computer software to refine the model so that the file is free from errors. The last stage is to gather the data. A 3D printer uses the revised model's exported Standard Tessellation Language (STL) to create the appropriate physical model. The materials are selected appropriately, and the printer settings are adjusted for a high-quality 3D printed model [8, 9].

4. Applications of 3D printing in dentistry

4.1 In the field of education

The digital imaging and scanning process is coupled with powerful software and 3D printing, causing drastic changes in training patterns and educational standards globally in the health sector, especially dentistry. Three-dimensional printing allows duplication of orofacial anatomy with high precision. Highly advanced 3D printers can reproduce jaws and hard and soft tissue images, which will be helpful for education training [10].

Dental students can thoroughly understand the anatomical model of the head and the surrounding area because the shape produced by 3D printing resembles the original shape. Siefert et al. and Chen et al., in their research comparing 3D printing models to cadaver models in education, concluded that 3D models could be an alternative model to replace cadavers in providing and training surgical practice for students who will perform oral maxillofacial surgery. Accurate 3D printed models help surgeons to research and train in a variety of different surgical techniques. These trainings can reduce operative time, avoid production errors, and increase surgical success [11, 12].

Apart from improving skills in performing surgery, these 3D printed models can also be used to teach pre-clinical students how to train for fixed prosthodontic treatment. This exercise can provide benefits so that students can practice making crown and veneer preparations. These 3D printing tooth models are made to resemble natural teeth and are perfect for preparation [10]. In the field of orthodontics and craniofacial cases, 3D print documentation is essential, and 3D prints can replace conventional prints. During training, real models from patients are beneficial for making orthodontic appliances, both removable and fixed [13].

For pre-clinical students who will carry out dental restorations, this 3D printing also helps students recognize tooth structure and techniques in carrying out cavity preparation. Training in endodontics can also influence prototyping speed. Endodontic training is carried out on teeth with ideal root canal conditions that are the same as the condition of the extracted original tooth. 3D printing can be obtained using scans of the patient obtained from CBCT, producing good results where the prints can be made before surgery (pre-surgical) and after endodontic surgery. This can help deal with problems encountered during surgery, such as bone prominence, morphological complications, root curves, and proximity to nerve bundles. 3D printing is also advantageous in teaching students and improving their perception of normal or complex root canals and the stages of preparation techniques with various root canals, such as access preparation and cleaning-shaping of root canals [14, 15].

In pediatric dentistry, this 3D printing can help students perform the SSC (stainless steel crown) technique. Models from patient radiographs can be used to visualize the pathological conditions that occur in terms of appearance, size, and depth of the caries lesion and the complexity of the tooth [16].

The use of 3D printing in the field of periodontics in education is beneficial in training, such as phantom heads, intra-oral examination of patients, and measurement of periodontal indices. Students can also use 3D printed models to experience the sensation of measurements such as pocket measurements, recession, and other periodontal examinations [7].

4.2 In the clinical field

3D printing in clinical care can be used for surgical guides, models, occlusal splints, and implants. In implant surgery, maxillary and mandibular reconstruction, orthognathic surgery, and temporomandibular joint surgery can be done with the help of 3D printing [13]. 3D printing can be used as a guide for surgery because it can help correct implant placement. Surgical guides have been successfully used in all single-tooth implant surgery types, including sinus lifting, whole oral cavity, and zygomatic implants [17]. Surgical guides such as cutting, drilling, and positioning guides are useful in mandibular and maxillary surgery and can help reduce operative time and improve clinical and esthetic results [18].

Models that are 3D printed and precisely depict the patient's anatomical state. The contour model represents a positive space model depicting the patient's anatomy. It is a 3D printed object that can be used for preoperative training on the model and osteosynthesis pre-forming/pre-bending or reconstruction plates according to planned results. When performing jaw surgery to align the mastication and occlusion in the correct position, the splint will be placed in the patient's mouth, replicating the location after surgery when the patient is in occlusion. This requires 3D printing designed with surgical software to match the condition [18, 19].

The application of 3D printing has resulted in a paradigm shift within the field of prosthodontics. Partial and fixed prostheses can be created without the hassle of a complete digital workflow involving scanning and printing. This digital prosthesis can be compared to conventional. The metal framework of removable partial prostheses can be obtained with excellent results and is easy to install. This causes errors to be eliminated, and this is related to laboratory procedures [20]. This condition aligns with the results of metallic full crowns and temporary acrylic crowns, which show good precision and margins when fitting compared to machined crowns. 3D printing can be used in ceramic restorations, molding, and other prosthodontic applications [21].

Recently, 3D printing has been used more frequently in orthodontics. Orthodontic appliances are made using CAD CAMs, intra-oral scans, and CBCT, with three-dimensional molding; ortho aligning can be done for crowded teeth. The use of occlusal splints with 3D techniques for TMJ disorders has been demonstrated by Salmi et al. [22] 3D printing can also be used in orthodontic brackets. The brackets are molded and adapted to the individual tooth surface. The bracket can be positioned accurately using 3D printing guides. Liu et al. use 3D printing of personalized arch-wire groove models to assist in giving the individual the appropriate archwire shape, and the process can be done easily and quickly. So, it can increase the effectiveness and perfection of manipulation and bending of wire arches. Additive manufacturing also allows various orthodontic devices, such as mouth guards, retainers, expanders, and apnea devices, to provide better intra-oral adaptation [23, 24].

3D printing in the field of endodontics is useful as a guide to cavity access, root canal treatment, and endosurgical procedures. In apical root canal lesions and calcified root canal conditions, a 3D printing model guide is also helpful in obtaining good results. Dimensional 3D printed guides used in root canal treatment can minimize measurement errors such as incorrect bur direction and root canal perforation, potentially hindering root canal treatment's success. The accuracy and precision of 3D-printed intra-coronal restorations are higher than conventional methods [7, 25].

Specific Implant patients use implants to repair defects in the cranio maxillofacial, which are related to cases of tumor, trauma, infection, or congenital deformity. This implant is made from polymer, titanium metal, and other compatible materials. During surgery, a mold is made of the patient's specific implant. This innovative technique has been used for many years for temporomandibular joint reconstruction and, more recently, for surgical rehabilitation in orthodontics [26]. 3D reconstruction of the skeletal frame on the contralateral (fit) side is used for mirroring. The main advantages are that this procedure replicates symmetrically in its use, is very accurate, and can predict the day after surgery. This is not only used on hard tissue but also on soft tissue that is planned to be placed [19].

In periodontal treatment cases, 3D printing can be used as a surgical guide to obtain zone esthetics in periodontal surgery. To obtain accuracy and precise treatment from gingival surgery, surgical template models are made with 3D printing. Besides, this mold can also help make scaffolds in regenerative periodontal surgery. The scaffold used can be obtained from 3D printing, namely bioprinting [7].

5. The role of 3D bioprinting in periodontal treatment

In dentistry, 3D printing has diverse applications and is a promising technology, potentially leading to new and exciting treatments. The use of 3D bioprinting technology for various applications has been proven to provide successful patient treatment options. Apart from rapid prototyping, currently, 3D printing can be used in various applications in dentistry, such as producing models and making scaffolds to help the periodontal regeneration process [27].

3D bioprinting is the first technology in the field of regenerative treatment that allows the creation of living tissue using living cells through a printing process. Periodontitis has become a more common disease among the public; thus, there is a need to increase periodontal regenerative procedures to restore normal periodontium for patients. Regenerative procedures require the placement of biocompatible tissue that is bioresorbable, supporting cell growth and proliferation in repairing the damage. Such structures can be created from 3D bioprinting technology that uses multiple bioinks and various bioprinting methods such as autonomous self-assembly, extrusion-based, and laser bioprinting to print tissue [1].

Imaging biomedical systems such as Cone Beam Computer Tomography is a valuable tool in the field of periodontics for diagnosing and better planning treatment by enabling visualization of disease, implant placement, and topography of the bone. Imaging CBCT provides scope for developing personalized scaffolding. CBCT topography data can be used to create a three-dimensional resolution image of the potential scaffolding, which can then be precisely erected over the damaged area. Three-dimensional printing has been applied to the development of polymer or ceramic scaffolds, as well as the creation of surgical guides and multiple scaffolding regeneration generations for clinical usage. A "system scaffolding bioactive" meant for network regeneration and repair can be created by combining this scaffolding technology with biological therapies or cells [28]. Periodontal tissue has a complex organization that requires the construction of multi-layered biomaterials to restore structural and functional integrity to the bone and periodontal ligament surfaces [29].

Periodontitis is an inflammatory disease caused by periodontal pathogens. The interaction of periodontal pathogens with host cells will affect the periodontium, causing tissue damage [7]. Damage that occurs to periodontal tissue will cause problems for the sufferer. Periodontal treatment is performed to treat and prevent further periodontal destruction. Periodontitis treatment aims to control inflammation through mechanical plaque removal and regenerate the periodontal. Conventional periodontitis treatment can only achieve long junctional epithelial attachments, so it cannot achieve total periodontal regeneration [30]. The need for treatment to achieve periodontal regeneration is increasing. Therefore, much clinical research is ongoing in 3D bioprinting to restore lost periodontal structures for individuals suffering from periodontitis. The periodontium structure has a quite complex morphology and requires special technical knowledge in the printing process [1].

Bioprinting is an advanced technology in the field of regeneration that facilitates tissue creation. Bioprinting is a technique used to design complex biological structures using bioinks. Before gaining insight into 3D bioprinting of the periodontium, it is important to understand the evolution of 3D bioprinting in the medical field [1, 4]. 3D bioprinting is a cutting-edge technology in the regeneration field facilitating multi-scale, biomimetic, multi-cellular tissue fabrication with highly complex tissue environments, intricate cytoarchitecture, structure–function hierarchy, and tissue-specific composition and mechanical properties [4]. As the term bioprinting implies, the process involves printing living tissue. This is done using a 3D *bioprinter* with a model designed on a computer. In this model, the *bioink* is coated through an additive manufacturing process to create tissue that imitates natural tissue [31].

6. Steps in 3D bioprinting

Several steps that are important to pay attention to in 3D Bioprinting are Pre-bioprinting: This step is the first step in the printing process, where the structure to be printed is designed and modeled as a 3D structure using Computed Tomography (CT) and MRI scanning. Every fine detail is recorded, and tomographic reconstruction is performed on the image to be printed in layers. Then, the bioink is prepared by isolation from living tissue and allowed to grow [7, 31]. The next step is bioprinting: in this process, bioinks are inserted into a printer cartridge, and based on a digital model, cells are accumulated in layers [32]. The post-bioprinting step involves maintaining the mechanical integrity and function of the 3D printing structure. In this step, tissue remodeling and growth are controlled by sending signals. More recently, the evolution of bioreactor technology has resulted in rapid tissue maturation, tissue vascularization, and increased transplant survival rates. The bioreactors differ depending on the tissue type [31, 33].

7. The role of bioprinting in periodontal regeneration

Periodontal tissue has a complex structure that requires multi-layered biomaterial construction to restore structural and functional integrity to the bone and ligament surfaces [7, 29]. Using additive biomanufacturing technology, periodontal regeneration may create hierarchical scaffolds that mirror the architectural characteristics and configurations of the periodontium, which is made up of hard and soft tissues including cementum, alveolar bone, periodontal ligament and gingiva. These scaffolds are called multiphasic constructs, as they have various compartments that recapitulate the original structure of the periodontal complex and are helpful in periodontal regeneration treatments [33, 34]. The main cells involved in periodontal regeneration are cement oblasts, osteoblasts, and periodontal fibroblasts. One source of renewable cells is stem cells. The several phases of periodontal regeneration include cell adhesion, migration, proliferation, and differentiation [35]. 3D printing innovation is a groundbreaking technology resulting in a paradigm shift in periodontal treatment. This helps in treatments such as installing dental implants, surgical guides, anatomical models, and so on, using computer-aided design data [7, 29].

Tissue engineering is one of the top areas of research interest in the medical field today. This process combines biological theory and engineering principles, helping injured tissue or organs recover and restore function through germ cells, biocompatible scaffolds, and bioactive factors [36]. Periodontal regeneration has been a research focus in oral tissue engineering for a long time. Guided tissue regeneration (GTR) is a common regeneration operation in periodontology [37].

The goal of regenerative tissue engineering is the regeneration of tissue and organs, either through the in vivo implantation of biomaterials in the form of grafts or the in vitro creation of replacement materials enriched with growth factors and cells, which are then transferred into the body at the defect site to promote regeneration. Tissue engineering is an interdisciplinary field encompassing stem cell biology, chemistry, materials science, medicine, and the production of biomaterials [38].

The environment surrounding periodontal defects can greatly influence the success rate of guided tissue regeneration (GTR), and biocompatible scaffolds provide a stable healing environment for periodontal tissue restoration. Therefore, making suitable scaffolding is very important. Due to the limited area of periodontal defects, constructing a scaffold appropriate to the size of the defect is challenging. Due to its high accuracy and efficiency, 3D bioprinting is becoming a new strategy. Existing 3D bioprinting methods are mainly divided into extrusion, droplet-jet bioprinting, and photocuring-based bioprinting [39]. When it comes to 3D bioprinting, bioink is unavoidable. The main material in 3D bioprinting is the composition of biocompatible materials, bioactive factors, and cells to create the final shape of the intended construction, determining the properties and biological features of the 3D bioprinting scaffold, which ultimately influences the results of periodontal tissue restoration [40].

A PCL (Polycaprolactone)—PGA (Polyglycolic Acid) scaffold created by manufacturing computers overcome these problems. This scaffold consists of special compartments of periodontal ligament and bone. Indirect 3D printing is used to create hybrid scaffolds. According to Park et al., to prepare the mold, the design of the pore size, channel orientation, and tissue-specific compartments is given great attention. Following fabrication, a PCL or PGA polymer solution is cast into the mold. Both compartments are combined with a thin layer of PCL to form a single scaffold. Mouse subcutaneous pockets were used to evaluate biomimetic random hybrid scaffolds for tooth and ligament surface engineering. They demonstrate the capacity for bone and periodontal ligament regeneration as well as the formation of parallel and obliquely oriented fibers. Adjustments were made to the design to simulate periodontal tissue better [41].

As an expansion of the biphasic scaffold, Lee et al. created the triphasic scaffold. Its goal is to incorporate different tissue regeneration. Using fused deposition modeling, the scaffold was made with compartments for the periodontal ligament, alveolar bone, and cementum/dentin contact. Biological cues and biophysical characteristics are anticipated to promote periodontal tissue regeneration. One design drawback of the PCL scaffold is its stiffness, which makes it challenging to adapt to the intricate 3D anatomy of different periodontal abnormalities [42].

Although 3D bioprinting technology has been available for many years, the high cost of 3D bioprinters, high energy consumption, operation and maintenance costs, clearance from ethical boards for using cells, and the requirement of trained operators have proven to be barriers to its development. Periodontal tissue engineering aims to use cells, scaffolds, and signaling molecules to restore the structure and functionality of both hard and soft tissues. The size of bone defects in periodontal disease varies, ranging from microscopic intraosseous flaws to massive horizontal and vertical bone defects that are significant in implant rehabilitation and periodontal healing [43]. For decades, efforts have been made to achieve predictable and reliable bone regeneration using various methods to improve the results of periodontal treatment.

Author details

Pitu Wulandari
Faculty of Dentistry, Universitas Sumatera Utara, Medan, Indonesia

*Address all correspondence to: pitu.wulandari@usu.ac.id

References

[1] Chandrasekharan T, Rajula MPB, Shankar PLR, Rajarajeswari. 3D bioprinting: Print the future of periodontics. Systematic Reviews in Pharmacy. 2021;**12**(8):477-483

[2] Dawood A, Marti BM, Sauret-Jackson V, Darwood A. 3D printing in dentistry. Nature Publication Group. 2015;**219**(11):521-529. DOI: 10.1038/sj.bdj.2015.914

[3] Berman B. 3-D printing: The new industrial revolution. Business Horizons. 2012;**55**:155-162. DOI: 10.1016/j.bushor.2011.11.003

[4] Vijayavenkataraman S, Yan W, Cheng, Lu WF, Wang CH, Fuh JYH. 3D bioprinting of tissue and organs for regenerative medicine. Advanced Drug Delivery Reviews. 2018;**132**:2-76. DOI: 10.1016/j.addr.2018.07.004

[5] Kohli TMA. 3D printing in dentistry—An overview. Acta Scientific Dental Sciences. 2019;**3**(6):35-41. DOI: 10.31080/ASDS.2019.03.0543

[6] Singh N, Sridevi N, Sawhny A. 3D Printing in Dentistry. Dentomed Publication House. 2021. pp. 1-107

[7] Shaikh SS, Nahar P, Shaikh SY, Sayed AJ, Habibullah MA. Current perspectives of 3D printing in dental applications. Brazilian Dental Science. 2021;(**July**):1-10. DOI: 10.14295/bds.2021.v24i3.2481

[8] Javaid M, Haleem A. Current status and applications of additive manufacturing in dentistry: A literature-based review. Journal of Oral Biology and Craniofacial Research. 2019:1-18. DOI: 10.1016/j.jobcr.2019.04.004

[9] Abdullah KA, Reed W. 3D printing in medical imaging and healthcare services. Journal of Medical Radiation Sciences. 2018:1-3. DOI: 10.1002/jmrs.292

[10] Kroger E, Dekiff M, Dirksen D. 3D printed simulation models based on real patient situations for hands-on practice. European Journal of Dental Education. 2016:1-7. DOI: 10.1111/eje.12229

[11] Seifert LB, Schnurr B, Herrera-Vizcaino C, et al. 3D-printed patient individualised models vs cadaveric models in an undergraduate oral and maxillofacial surgery curriculum: Comparison of student's perceptions. European Journal of Dental Education. 2020;**24**:799-806. DOI: 10.1111/eje.12522

[12] Chen S, Pan Z, Wu Y, et al. The role of three-dimensional printed models of skull in anatomy education: A randomized controlled trail. Scientific Reports. 2017:1-11. DOI: 10.1038/s41598-017-00647-1

[13] Oberoi G, Nitsch S, Edelmayer M, Janjic K, Muller AS, Agis H. 3D printing—Encompassing the facets of dentistry. Frontiers in Bioengineering and Biotechnology. 2018;**6**:1-13. DOI: 10.3389/fbioe.2018.00172

[14] Shah P, Chong BS. 3D imaging, 3D printing and 3D virtual planning in endodontics. Clinical Oral Investigations. 2018:16-18

[15] Soares CJ, Raposo LHA, Soares PV, et al. Effect of different cements on the biomechanical behavior of teeth restored with cast dowel-and-cores—In vitro and FEA analysis. Journal of Prosthodontics. 2010;**19**:130-137. DOI: 10.1111/j.1532-849X.2009.00527.x

[16] Mathieu M, Alice B, Jean-Noel V, Frederic V. Comparison of student's

perceptions between 3D printed models versus series models in pediatric dentistry hands-on session. European Journal of Dental Education. 2018:1-14. DOI: 10.1111/eje.12404

[17] Rinaldi M, Ganz SD. Computer-guided approach for placement of zygomatic implants: Novel protocol and surgical guide. The Compendium of Continuing Education in Dentistry. 2019;**40**(6):e1-e9. Available from: http://www.ncbi.nlm.nih.gov/pubmed/30829495

[18] Ghai S, Sharma Y, Jain N, Satpathy M, Pillai AK. Use of 3-D printing technologies in craniomaxillofacial surgery: A review. Oral and Maxillofacial Surgery. 2018:1-14. DOI: 10.1007/s10006-018-0704-z

[19] Louvrier A, Marty P, Weber E, et al. How useful is 3D printing in Maxillo-facial surgery. Journal of Stomatology, Oral and Maxillofacial Surgery. 2017;**17**:1-18. DOI: 10.1016/j.jormas.2017.07.002

[20] Hu F, Pei Z, Wen Y. Using intraoral scanning technology for three-dimensional printing of Kennedy class I removable partial denture metal framework: A clinical report. Journal of Prosthodontics. 2017:1-4. DOI: 10.1111/jopr.12712

[21] Katreva I, Dikova T, Abadzhiev M, et al. 3D-printing in comtemporary prosthodontic treatment. Scripta Scientifica Medicinae Dentalis. 2016;**2**(1):7-11. DOI: 10.14748/ssmd.v1i1.1446

[22] Salmi M, Paloheimo KS, Tuomi J, Ingman T, Mäkitie A. A Digital Process for Additive Manufacturing of Occlusal Splints: A Clinical Pilot Study. Apr 2013. pp. 1-6. DOI: 10.1098/rsif.2013.0203

[23] Liu G, Qin H, Zhen H, Liu B, Wang X, Tao X. 3D printing of personalized archwire groove model for orthodontics: Design and implementation. International Journal of Advanced Computer Science and Applications. 2018;**9**(12):37-41

[24] Jheon AH, Oberoi S, Solem RC, Kapila S. Moving towards precision orthodontics: An evolving paradigm shift in the planning and delivery of customized orthodontic therapy. Orthodontics & Craniofacial Research. 2017;**20**(March):106-113. DOI: 10.1111/ocr.12171

[25] Garcia-sanchez A, Mainkar A, Ordonez E, Sanchez S, Weinstein G. 3D-printed guide for endodontic surgery. Clinical Dentistry Review. 2019;**3**(13):2-7. DOI: 10.1007/s41894-019-0048-6

[26] Huang MF, Alfi D, Alfi J, Huang AT. The use of patient-specific implants in oral and maxillofacial surgery. Oral and Maxillofacial Surgery Clinics of North America. 2019;**31**:593-600

[27] Patel R, Sheth T, Shah S, Shah M. A New Leap in Periodontics: Three-Dimensional (3D) Printing. 2017;**8**(1&2):1-7. DOI: 10.1177/2229411217729102

[28] Rasperini G, Pilipchuk SP, Flanagan CL, et al. 3D-printed bioresorbable scaffold for periodontal repair. Journal of Dental Research. 2015;**94**(June):1-5. DOI: 10.1177/0022034515588303

[29] Vaquette C, Pilipchuk SP, Bartold PM, Hutmacher DW, Giannobile WV, Ivanovski S. Tissue engineered constructs for periodontal regeneration: Current status and future perspectives. Advanced Healthcare Materials. 2018:1-20. DOI: 10.1002/adhm.201800457

[30] Deas DE, Moritz AJ, Sagun RS, Gruwell SF, Powell CA. Scaling and root planing vs. conservative surgery in the treatment of chronic periodontitis. Periodontology 2000. 2016;**17**:128-139. DOI: 10.1111/prd.12114

[31] Murphy SV, Atala A. 3D bioprinting of tissues and organs. Nature Biotechnology. 2014;**32**(8):773-785. DOI: 10.1038/nbt.2958

[32] Ozbolat IT. Bioprinting scale-up tissue and organ constructs for transplantation. Trends in Biotechnology. 2015:1-6. DOI: 10.1016/j.tibtech.2015.04.005

[33] Obregon F, Vaquette C, Hutmacher DW, Bertassoni LE. Three-dimensional bioprinting for regenerative dentistry and craniofacial tissue engineering. JDR Clinical Research Supplement. 2015;(X):1S-11S. DOI: 10.1177/0022034515588885

[34] Ivanovski S, Vaquette C, Gronthos S, Hutmacher DW, Bartold PM. Multhiphasic scaffolds for periodontal tissue engineering. Journal of Dental Research. 2016;(**January**):1212-1221. DOI: 10.1177/0022034514544301

[35] Lakkaraju RB, Guntakandla VR, Gooty JR, Palaparthy RB, Vundela RK, Bommireddy V. Three-dimensional printing—A new vista for periodontal regeneration: A review. International Journal of Medical Reviews. 2017;**4**(3):81-85. DOI: 10.29252/ijmr-040305.Introduction

[36] Tatullo M, Marrelli M, Paduano F. The regenerative medicine in oral and maxillofacial surgery: The Most important innovations in the clinical application of mesenchymal stem cells. International Journal of Medical Sciences. 2015;**12**(1):72-77. DOI: 10.7150/ijms.10706

[37] Nuñez J, Vignoletti F, Caffesse RG, Sanz M. Cellular therapy in periodontal regeneration. Periodontology 2000. 2019;**79**:107-116. DOI: 10.1111/prd.12250

[38] Cremers NAJ, Suttorp M, Gerritsen MM, et al. Mechanical stress changes the complex interplay between HO-1, inflammation and fibrosis, during excisional wound repair. Frontiers in Medicine. 2015:1-13

[39] Raveau S, Jordana F. Tissue engineering and three printing in periodontal regeneration: A literature review. Journal of Clinical Medicine. 2020:1-21

[40] D'Avanzo N, Bruno MC, Giudice A, et al. Influence of materials properties on bio-physical features and effectiveness of 3D-scaffolds for periodontal regeneration. Molecules. Mar 2021;**26**(6):2-30. DOI: 10.3390/molecules26061643

[41] Park CH, Rios HF, Jin Q, et al. Biomimetic hybrid scaffolds for engineering human tooth- ligament interfaces. Biomaterials. 2010:1-7. DOI: 10.1016/j.biomaterials.2010.04.027. Biomimetic

[42] Lee CH, Hajibandeh J, Suzuki T, Fan A, Shang P, Mao JJ. Three-dimensional printed multiphase scaffolds for regeneration of periodontium complex. Tissue Engineering. Part A. 2014;**20**:1342-1351. DOI: 10.1089/ten.tea.2013.0386

[43] Kahl M, Gertig M, Hoyer P, Friedrich O, Gilbert DF. Ultra-low-cost 3D bioprinting: Modification and application of an off-the-shelf desktop 3D-printer for biofabrication. Frontiers in Bioengineering and Biotechnology. 2019;(**July**):1-12. DOI: 10.3389/fbioe.2019.00184

Chapter 4

Non-Invasive Periodontal Evaluations with the Novel Gingivitis Extent and Gingivitis Severity Indices

Fowziya M. Ali

Abstract

The periodontium serves as the dentition's base. It connects the tooth to the alveolar socket, permits sensations, and aids in supporting and shielding the tooth. In youngsters, gingivitis and periodontitis are typically curable and reversible diseases that should be identified early and treated right away. To precisely document these disorders and determine the effectiveness or failure of treatment, suitable clinical indices must be accessible. Gingivitis in children can appear in a variety of ways, and it has been observed that these manifestations get worse with age and peak during puberty. The majority of adult periodontal disease consequences can be attributed to early life experiences. Numerous systemic or local contributory variables cause children's gingival disease. Concern about medical conditions, place of examination, and age of children are the main determining factors in the selection of an appropriate index for use in critically or at-risk children. The use of the novel gingival extent (GE) and gingival severity (GS) indices to assess periodontal disease as a modification of the PMA index enlightens that such indices are non-invasive, simple, and thought to be suitable.

Keywords: non-invasive GE and GS indices, periodontal disease index, critically and at-risk children, gingivitis, gingivitis severity scoring

1. Introduction

The 2018 World Workshop of the American Academy of Periodontology (AAP) and the European Federation of Periodontology (EFP) defined periodontal health as lacking clinically detectable inflammation [1]. This AAP/EFP definition is mostly determined by bleeding on probing BOP scores and probing pocket depth PPD. The features of a healthy periodontium are that the gingiva is typically coral pink but may vary due to physiologic pigmentation among some races, whereas the alveolar mucosa is deep red. The texture of the gingiva varies with age and is typically smooth in youth, stippled in adulthood, and again becomes smoother with advanced age. Stippled tissue has a texture similar to the rind of an orange, and the gingival margin is several millimetres coronal to the cemento-enamel junction (CEJ). On a tooth that has fully erupted, the gingival sulcus may be 0.5–3 mm deep. The alveolar crest in teenagers with a healthy periodontium is 0.4–1.9 mm apical to the CEJ [2]. However, it was found that until the teeth reach occlusion, the gingival sulcus for all tooth types falls from 3.09–2.86 to 2.00–2.20 mm during the eruption period [3]. A flexible measuring strip measured the gingival sulcus at six mesio-buccal (MB) and six bucco-cervical (BC) locations six times over 20 weeks. The results showed that the PD scored 0.5 to 4.5 mm, which varied significantly between patients with different sites [4]. As seen in **Figure 1**, the periodontal probe is used to evaluate the depth of the gingival sulcus surrounding the tooth.

On the other hand, a periodontal probe is used to measure bleeding index, pocket depths, and keratinized gingiva width.

Periodontal probing should only be done on teeth that are completely erupted.

A well-maintained sulcular depth of no more than 3 mm can be easily cleaned with a toothbrush and other oral hygiene products [5].

Among the most prevalent oral conditions affecting dentate individuals, periodontal infections are known to lead to tooth loss [6–10].

Epidemiological studies of periodontal diseases commonly start with the study of the prevalence and incidence of the disease. After the disease's scope and distribution have been examined, the information that is now available can be used to research the disease's nature and aetiological variables, and help, planning for future resource allocation is aided by understanding how the illness impacts society and the economy [11, 12]. There are several gingival indices developed which rely upon bleeding following 'gentle probing' such as Russell's periodontal index, sulcular bleeding index (SBI), papillary bleeding index (PBI), gingival index (GI), and Löe and Silness and their modifications [12–16]. However, Lobene's modification of the Löe and Silness gingiva index method is non-invasive but depends upon using posterior teeth [15, 16]. Moreover, based on the existence or absence of bleeding, the World Health Organization (WHO) created the Community Periodontal Index for Treatment Needs (CPITN) in 1982 [17].

However, some authors have questioned the usefulness of bleeding as the most sensitive sign of gingivitis, pointing out that in the early stages of the condition, colour and contour changes have been seen to occur before bleeding on probing [12, 14]; see **Figure 2**.

Following the 2001 Policy Statement of the British Society of Periodontology (BSP) regarding the diagnosis and treatment of periodontal disease in adults receiving primary dental care, as well as the 2011 revisions to the BSP's "Referral Policy and

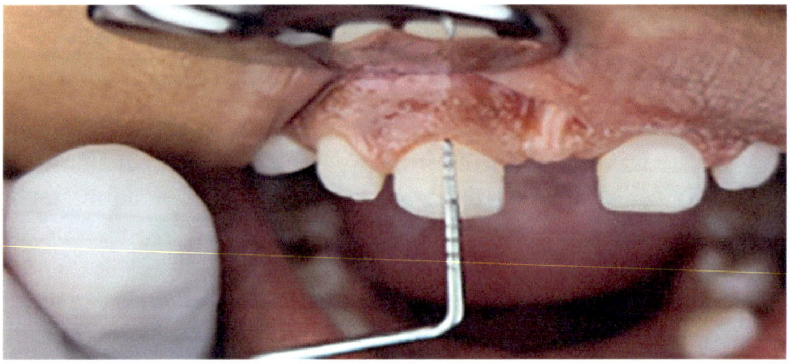

Figure 1.
Measurements of gingival sulcular depth and bleeding that are employed by the majority of periodontal indices that are currently available.

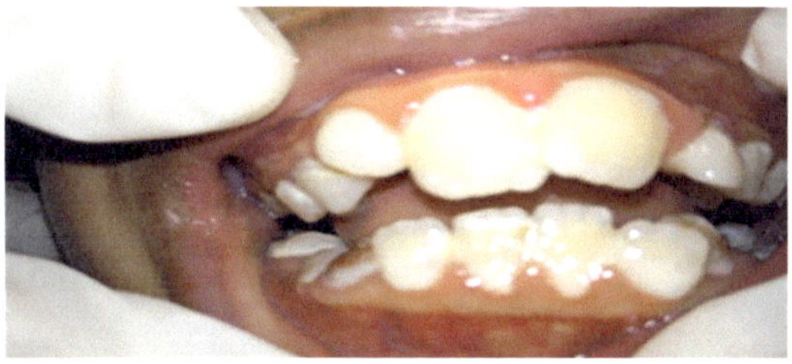

Figure 2.
A change in the colour and shape of the gingival tissues indicates the presence of gingivitis.

Parameters of Care" and "Basic Periodontal Examination" documents [15, 16, 18–20]. It is acknowledged that similar standards regarding children and adolescents are necessary. The British Society of Paediatric Dentistry (BSPD) and the British Society of Periodontology and Implant Dentistry (BSP) continue to emphasize the significance of periodontal screening for children in conjunction with the release of updated national guidelines for the treatment of patients under the age of 18 in primary care settings. It is clear with the BSP's original adult guidelines materials (www.bsperio.org.uk). Furthermore, according to the 1999 International Workshop for Classification of Periodontal Diseases and Conditions, children and adolescents can be affected by a wide variety of periodontal diseases including endodontic lesions-related periodontitis, abscesses of the periodontium, necrotizing periodontal diseases, aggressive periodontitis, chronic periodontitis and gingival disorders.

Dental professionals play a crucial role in the early detection and diagnosis of periodontal and gingival disorders. By doing this, the primary dental care environment will have the best opportunity to provide successful treatment or relevant speciality services will be referred to.

Management needs to incorporate effective oral hygiene practices in childhood and adolescence, which should extend into early adulthood and beyond [21, 22]:

However, one of the issues with probing is the amount of pressure the examiner can apply; even with light probing, some examiners have been known to apply pressures as high as 130 g [21]. In addition, if the probing force is more than 25 g, the gingiva may become injured and further bleeding may happen [22]. Additionally, it has been shown that while a 15-minute gap between the first and subsequent probes may lower the risk, repeated probing may make bleeding more likely [22].

The following guidelines for an efficient index for the study of periodontal disease [16, 23, 24]:

1. An index should be easy to use and cost as little time and money as possible.

2. The criteria that define the index must be understandable and clear.

3. The index should indicate the clinical phases of the disease with equivalent sensitivity across its range.

4. The index should be possible to evaluate the index statistically.

5. The precision, accuracy, validity, and reliability of the measurements obtained using the gingival index must also be taken into account when choosing the index for a clinical trial.

6. Since an index needs to reasonably accurately identify the severity of the condition, it should be quantitative.

7. It must be appropriate for statistical analysis.

2. Methodology

The condition of the periodontal tissues will be evaluated using a contemporary, non-invasive method that the researcher has created.

Probing of the gingiva should not be used. A hygienic mouth mirror or wooden tongue blade may be used to retract the lips, and excellent lighting is required. The patient can be examined in bed or on the couch for a simple oral examination.

2.1 The GE index

A modification of the PMA index was used to assess the prevalence of gingivitis [25, 26]. Both the anterior and posterior segments of both arches were studied in these investigations. The next claim was that, in any given month, the ten anterior teeth—which could serve as index teeth, as shown in **Figures 3** and **4**—represented a significant majority of the gingivitis observed in the front teeth's anterior region.

The procedure was based on visually assessing the presence or absence of the inflammation in three parts of the gingiva. Changes in gingival colour (redness), oedema, loss of stippling, increased gingival crevicular fluid flow, engorgement, bleeding, and, in rare instances, ulceration are among the clinical indicators of gingivitis [1, 2, 15].

The following were the three separate zones examined:

1. Papillary (P), the area of the gingiva that fills the gap between two adjacent teeth in the interdental space.

2. Marginal (M), is the area of gingiva that surrounds the tooth's neck in the form of a collar of free gingiva.

3. Attached (A), is that part of the gingiva which is attached by a dense fibrous tissue to the underlying bone.

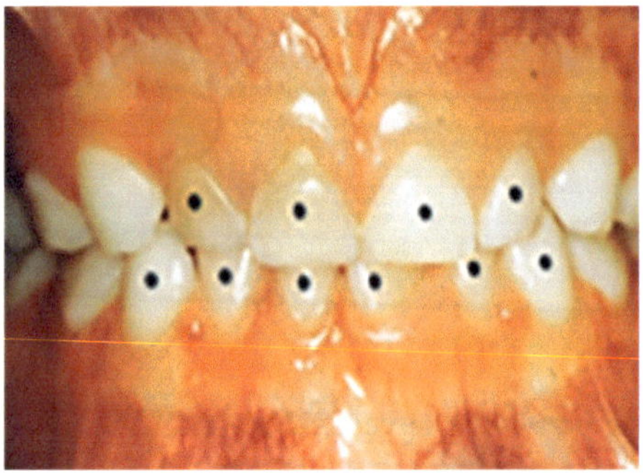

Figure 3.
Four primary upper incisors and six lower anterior teeth comprise the index teeth for primary dentition.

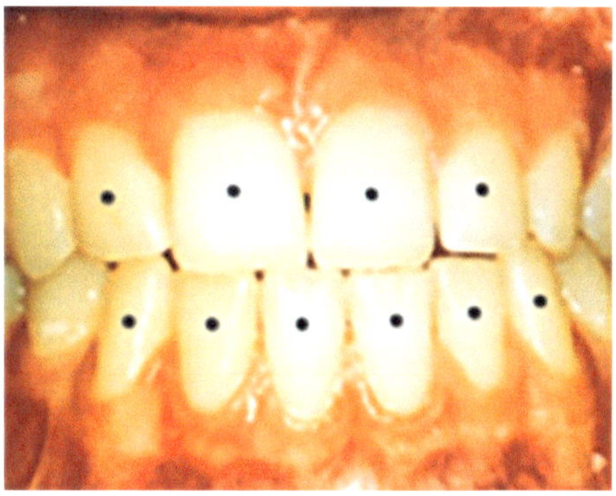

Figure 4.
Four permanent upper incisors and six lower anterior teeth comprise the index teeth for permanent dentition.

Gingivitis extent scores (GE)	Number of inflamed units
GE 1	No inflammation within the units
GE 2	Scores for inflamed units (1–6).
GE 3	Scores ranging from 7 to 14 inflamed units.
GE 4	Results for the inflamed units (15–18).

Table 1.
Distribution of gingivitis extent (GE) scores.

The score for each subject was computed as the sum of the numbers of all examined areas in both arches. For analysis, the subjects were divided into four groups of gingivitis extent scores as shown in **Table 1**.

For the presentation of results, the gingivitis extent scores will be abbreviated as GE1, GE2, GE3, and GE4.

The index teeth used were the four upper incisors and the six lower anterior teeth from cuspid to cuspid. This includes three papillae and four margins in upper index teeth and five papillae and six margins in lower index teeth.

The number of papillae on the maxillary arch affected by gingivitis (P) out of the papillae between lateral and central incisors and between central incisors was recorded (maximum number 3). The number of affected margins (M) was recorded (maximum 4 for all incisors), as was the number of affected sites of attached gingiva (A) (maximum 4 for all incisors). A similar process was carried out for the lower arch, which encompassed the lower canines and incisors, and five papillae, six margins and six zones of attached gingivae were examined.

For descriptive purposes and statistical analysis, the gingivitis extent (GE) should be divided into the following in **Table 1**.

3. Gingivitis severity (GS) scoring

The evaluation was based solely on appearance to the naked eye, and the degree of inflammation was quantitatively rated in steps of increasing intensity and extent.

Gingivitis severity (GS) scores	Features that are typical of the degree of severity of gingivitis.
GS0	Absence of the following symptoms indicative of gingivitis: Colour: light pink; texture: solid, with no bleeding under strong digital pressure.
GS1	Mild inflammation accompanied by a tiny change in colour and minimal contour loss.
GS2	Moderate inflammation is characterised by redness, glazing, and swelling. The margins or papillae seem rounded.
GS3	Severe inflammation accompanied by increased redness, swelling, and sporadic bleeding. Mild ulceration may be observed.
GS4	Exceedingly severe, including ulcers and sloughing.

Table 2.
Gingivitis severity (GS) scores and the characteristic features.

A severity score for gingivitis was assigned to each subject based on the mean of scores from both maxillary and mandibular arches of the most severely affected papilla, margin, or zone of attached gingiva, as shown in **Table 2**.

4. Discussion

Clinical periodontal evaluations should be routinely recorded and diagnosed as part of children and adolescent dental exams. An oral examination and an initial assessment should comprise an assessment of the soft and hard tissues and a basic description of periodontal health. It is important to record any abnormal gingival colour, shape, oedema, and the presence and location of the inflammation [27–31]. Even while tooth plaque is the primary aetiological agent of periodontal disease, a person's reaction to plaque formation can be altered by several systemic and local factors (risk factors), which can also affect how quickly gingivitis progresses to periodontitis. Gingivitis caused by plaque may occur at any age, starting early childhood and continuing through adolescence and beyond. Based on studies in the field of epidemiology, the prevalence of gingivitis is low in preschoolers, but it gradually rises and peaks around puberty. This could be because of changes in the bacterial makeup of dental plaque, alterations in the inflammatory cell response, and hormonal changes [32]. The accumulation of supragingival plaque causes an inflammatory cell infiltrate in the gingival connective tissue. It disrupts the attachment of the junctional epithelium, allowing the plaque to migrate apically and deepen the gingival sulcus. This process is the cause of plaque-induced gingivitis. Severe inflammation can also cause gingival swelling, which deepens the false gingival pocket. The most apical extent of the junctional epithelium is still at the CEJ, and there has been no periodontal loss of attachment [33–35]. This process is completely reversible with effective plaque removal. The 2003 Child Dental Health Survey involved a representative sample of 5-, 8-, 12-, and 15-year-olds in the United Kingdom, and 10,381 children were examined, and the results showed that the 8- and 12-year-olds had higher levels of gingival inflammation and plaque than the younger cohort. In the epidemiological survey, gingival inflammation was present in only approximately one-third of 5-year-olds, compared to two-thirds of 8- and 12-year-old children and half of 15-year-olds [36]. Several studies have shown that, under the best of circumstances, routinely and carefully removing dental plaque can stop the development of early periodontal disease [37–41].

Individuals may also present with non-plaque-induced gingival lesions, several of which should be referred. While one of the most prevalent inflammatory diseases in humans is plaque-induced gingivitis, there are some of less common but frequently very significant non-plaque-induced gingival illnesses. The non-plaque-induced gingival lesions can be pathologic alterations restricted to the gingival tissues, but they are also frequently signs of systemic disorders. Based on the aetiology of the lesions, a classification is suggested, which consists of the following: traumatic lesions; endocrine, nutritional, and metabolic diseases; specific infections; inflammatory and immune conditions and lesions; reactive processes; neoplasms; and genetic/developmental disorders [42, 43]. The use of a Simplified Basic Periodontal Examination BPE to assess periodontal needs should be started at 7 years of age on six index teeth in all co-operative children and adolescents [30, 44–47]. However, periodontal screening with a simplified BPE index is not suitable for hospitalized, medically unfit or at-risk patients because it depends on gingival probing. In addition, screening for gingival diseases is not suitable for children less than seven. Children under the age of seven, those whose anterior primary and permanent teeth have fully erupted, and both cooperative and non-cooperative children can all benefit from using the GE and GS indices. It is more convenient and non-invasive for children who are at risk or in the hospital because it does not require probing, costly equipment, or revealing solutions.

In addition, the GE and GS indices are quicker and easier to use than the Simplified Basic Periodontal Examination in identifying periodontal problems in adults and children under the age of seven. In order to apply the required therapeutic and preventative measures, a reliable diagnosis can be made without the need for additional probing.

Accurate diagnosis and appropriate treatment and prevention strategies can only be implemented when periodontal diseases are detected early in both children and adults. However, there are certain difficulties with screening for periodontal disease in children, including cooperation (in the case of very young children) and increased probing depths (false pockets) related to partially erupted teeth and the mixed dentition stage. Three groups of children and teenagers, ages 7, 12 and 17, were examined for the existence of genuine and false pockets, with and without gingival haemorrhage on probing. When the first molars and incisors erupted, false pockets were common around the age of seven. By the age of 12, they had considerably decreased, and by 17, they were virtually non-existent. Even at 17 years old, false pockets continued to be an issue around the second molars [48]. There are restrictions when using a periodontal probe, and various variables could affect the results. These could include elements about the time, shape, and characteristics of each type of probe, such as the marking interval accuracy, probe thickness, probe angulation, probing force, reference point accuracy, subgingival obstruction, root anatomy, tissue condition at the deepest pocket's depth, and any pain brought on by probing [49–53]. The third-generation probes have several drawbacks as well, such as a diminished ability to perceive and touch the operator. Furthermore, the accuracy of the measurement may be impacted by an increase in the patient's discomfort and the gingival tissue's state of inflammation. Thus, for every generation of probes, the probe's efficiency needs to be assessed. Third-generation probes seem to be more useful, but because of their low efficiency, their application is essentially limited to research. A study conducted by Perry et al. used Ramfjord teeth *in vitro* as a part of an in vivo study to determine the clinical importance of different types of probes, whether probing a healthy periodontium or in maintenance patients. When these researchers probed a healthy subject, they found no clinically significant differences between the types of probes [54].

It would be better to assess periodontal diseases by using the GE index to allow the enumeration of inflamed units in the anterior segment of the four upper maxillary teeth and lower six anterior teeth safely, quickly, time-saving, easily and more accurately rather than recording posterior teeth It could be more accessible and accurate to record the anterior teeth as an index than the posterior teeth. Recording the anterior teeth as an index would be more accessible and precise than the posterior. Therefore, uniformity in observations could be achieved, leading to more meaningful comparisons.

Although many studies have been conducted to assess periodontal disease in physically healthy children based on probing and extensive measurements such as radiographic interpretation, there is a need to assess the periodontal health in critically ill, hospitalized, and at-risk children. The GE index is useful, simple, safe, and non-invasive based on visual examination of four anterior maxillary and six anterior mandibular teeth. In addition to the enumeration of inflamed units by (GE index), there is further assessment of the degree of inflammation (severity of gingival inflammation) by gingivitis severity index (GS) whereby a score is assigned to the most inflamed unit. The severity score for the patient was expressed as a mean of both the anterior maxillary and mandibular indexed teeth [29].

The limitation of these indices is that it is not possible to diagnose the attachment loss from these indices.

5. Conclusions

Both indices demonstrated non-invasiveness, easiness, high quantitively, fast, increased accessibility in visible places and lack of usage of sharp equipment. Both cooperative and non-cooperative patients can employ this method, including patients with disabilities and health issues.

Examining periodontal disease in critically ill, hospitalized, and at-risk severely disabled people is appropriate when using both the new GE and GS indexes. The majority of children and adults need periodontal screening using non-invasive modern GE and GS methods in dental offices, community settings, and hospitals.

6. Recommendations

Guidelines by ©2012 British Society of Periodontology and The British Society of Paediatric Dentistry [55].

1. Practicing good dental hygiene and mechanical plaque removal [22]. It offers extra advantages in terms of lowering the risk of dental caries. Adherence to the Department of Health Guidelines on Promoting Better Oral Health is recommended (2009) [23].

2. They are advised to start brushing as soon as the first primary tooth appears.

3. For the best caries control, patients over the age of 3 should use a family toothpaste (1350–1500 ppm fluoride), while children under the age of 3 should use toothpaste with at least 1000 ppm fluoride.

4. Sufficient parental monitoring is necessary for younger children.

5. The clinician should stress the importance of thoroughly cleaning all tooth surfaces, as no toothbrushing approach is superior to another.

6. To do this, the patient's current toothbrushing method might need to be adjusted. Tablet disclosure is known to assist in identifying areas that are being ignored.

Author details

Fowziya M. Ali
Paediatric Dentistry Department, University of Benghazi, Benghazi, Libya

*Address all correspondence to: fowziya.ali@uob.edu.ly

References

[1] Chapple IL, Mealey BL, Van Dyke TE, Bartold PM, Dommisch H, Eickholz P, et al. Periodontal health and gingival diseases and conditions on an intact and a reduced periodontium: Consensus report of workgroup 1 of the 2017 world workshop on the classification of periodontal and peri-implant diseases and conditions. Journal of Periodontology. 2018;**89**:S74-S84

[2] Hausmann E, Allen K, Clerehugh V. What alveolar crest level on a bitewing radiograph represents bone loss? Journal of Periodontology. 1991;**62**:570-572

[3] Mitova N, Rashkova M. Depth of gingival sulcus in healthy children with erupting permanent teeth. Folia Medica. 2020;**62**(2):302-307. DOI: 10.3897/folmed.62.e47567

[4] Smith RG, Çakici S, Newcombe RG. Variations in the clinical sulcus depth of healthy human gingiva: A longitudinal study. Journal of Periodontal Research. 1996;**31**(3):181-186

[5] Valerie C, Kindelan S. Guidelines produced in conjunction with the British society of periodontology and implant dentistry and British society of paediatric dentistry updated September 2021. Assessment and management of the periodontal condition in children (bsperio.org.uk) ©2021 British society of periodontology and implant dentistry and British society of paediatric dentistry

[6] Maguire A, Rugg-Gunn AJ, Butler TJ. Dental health of children taking antimicrobial and non-antimicrobial liquid oral medications long-term. Caries Research. 1996;**30**:16-21

[7] Ettinger RL. Epidemiology of dental caries. A broad review. Dental Clinics of North America. 1999;**43**(4):679-694

[8] PHSPS, Public Health Service. Healthy people 2000. In: Progress Report on Oral Health. Washington, DC: U.S. Department of Health and Human Services. 1995-1996. p. 1995

[9] Petersen EP. The world oral health report continuous improvement of oral health in the 21st century–The approach of the WHO global oral health programme. Community Dentistry and Oral Epidemiology. 2003;**31**(1):3-24

[10] Moynihan P, Petersen PE. Diet, nutrition and the prevention of dental diseases. Public Health Nutrition. 2004;**7**(1A):201-226

[11] CDC. Principles of epidemiology in public health practice: An introduction to applied epidemiology and biostatistics. [online]. 2006 [Accessed: September 2, 2020]

[12] Greenstein G. The role of bleeding upon probing in the diagnosis of periodontal disease. Journal of Periodontology. 1984;**55**:684-686

[13] Russell AL. The periodontal index. Journal of Periodontology. 1967;**38**(6P2):585-591. DOI: 10.1902/jop.1967.38.6_part2.585. Available from: europepmc.org

[14] Bollmer BW, Sturzenberger OP, Lehnhoff RW, Bosma ML, Lang NP, Mallatt ME, et al. A comparison of three clinical indices for measuring gingivtitis. Journal of Clinical Periodontology. 1986;**13**:392-395

[15] Lobene RR. Discussion: Current status of indices for measuring gingivitis. Journal of Clinical Periodontology. 1986;**13**:381-382

[16] Lobene RR, Mankodi SM, Ciancio SG, Lamm RA, Charles CH, e Ross NM. Correlations among gingival indices: A methodology study. Journal of Periodontology. 1989;**60**(3):159-162

[17] Croxson LJ. The origins and development of the Community Periodontal Index of Treatment Needs. The New Zealand Dental Journal. 1998;**94**:118-120

[18] British Society of Periodontology. Periodontology in general dental practice in the United Kingdom. A policy statement. 2001. Available from: https://www.bsperio.org.uk

[19] British Society of Periodontology. Basic periodontal examination (BPE). 2011. Available from: https://www.bsperio.org.uk

[20] British Society of Periodontology. Referral policy and parameters of care updated 2011. Available from: https://www.bsperio.org.uk

[21] Armitage GC. Development of a classification system for periodontal diseases and conditions. Annals of Periodontology. 1999;**4**(1):1-6

[22] Clerehugh V, Tugnait A. Treatment Planning: Periodontal Problems in Children and Adolescents. Churchill's Textbook of Periodontics. Practical Periodontics - Google Books; 2015

[23] Hazen SP. Indices for the measurement of gingival inflammation in clinical studies of oral hygiene and periodontal disease. Journal of Periodontal Research. 1974;**9**:61-77

[24] Ramfjord S. Indices for prevalence and incidence of periodontal disease. Journal of Periodontology. 1959;**30**:51-59

[25] Massler M, Rosenberg H, Carter W, Schour I. Gingivitis in young adult males: Lack of effectiveness of a permissive programme of toothbrushing. Journal of Periodontology. 1957;**28**:111-124

[26] Massler M, Schour I, Chopra B. Occurrence of gingivitis in suburban Chicago school children. Journal Periodontology. 1950;**21**:146-164

[27] Van der Weijden GA, van Loveren C. Mechanical plaque removal in step-1 of care. Periodontology 2000. Wiley Online Library. 2023;**00**:1-17. DOI: 10.1111/prd.12541

[28] Godson J, Gallagher J. Delivering better oral health 2021-What's new and where next. Community Dental Health. 2021;**38**(4):224-225

[29] Ali FM, Najm M. Investigation of the periodontal health status of group Libyan children using a novel gingivitis extent and severity indices: With reference to microbial gingival pathogens. Middle East Journal of Applied Sciences. 2019;**9**(4):901-905

[30] Cole E, Ray-Chaudhuri A, Vaidyanathan M, Johnson J, Sood S. Simplified basic periodontal examination (BPE) in children and adolescents: A guide for general dental practitioners. Dental Update. 2014;**41**(4):328-337

[31] Kumar A, Masamatti SS, Virdi MS. Periodontal diseases in children and adolescents: A clinician's perspective part 2. Dental Update. 2012;**39**(9):639-652

[32] Bimstein E, Matsson L. Growth and development considerations in the diagnosis of gingivitis and periodontitis in children. Pediatric Dentistry. 1999;**21**:186-191

[33] Murakami S, Mealey BL, Mariotti A, Chapple IL. Dental plaque–induced gingival conditions. Journal of Clinical Periodontology. 2018;**45**:S17-S27

[34] Preethanath RS, Ibraheem WI, Anil A. Pathogenesis of gingivitis. Oral Diseases. Feb 1975;**3**(1):1-4

[35] Clerehugh V, Tugnait A, Milward MR, Chapple IL. Periodontology at a Glance. John Wiley & Sons; 2024. Available from: nih.gov

[36] Bosnak A, Jorgić-Srdjak K, Marcević T, Plancak D. The width of the clinically-defined keratinized gingival in the mixed dentition. ASDC Journal of Dentistry for Children. 2002;**69**:266-270

[37] Badersten A, Egelberg J, Koch G. Effect of monthly prophlaxis on caries and gingivitis in school children. Community Dentistry and Oral Epidemiology. 1975;**3**:1-4

[38] Axelsson P, Lindhe J. The effect of a plaque control programme on gingivitis and dental caries in school children. Journal of Dental Research. 2005;**6**:31. DOI: 10.1038/sj.ebd.6400325.pdf

[39] Agerbaek N, Paulsen S, Nelson B, Glavind L. Effect of professional tooth-cleaning every third week on gingivitis and dental caries in children. Community Dentistry and Oral Epidemiology. 1977;**6**:40-41

[40] Hamp SE, Lindhe J, Farrell J, Johansson LA, Karlsson R. Effect of a field programme based on systematic plaque control on caries and gingivitis in school children after three years. Community Dentistry and Oral Epidemiology. 1978;**6**:17-23

[41] Hausen H. Oral health promotion reduces plaque and gingival bleeding in the short term. Evidence-Based Dentistry. 2005;**6**:31

[42] Holmstrup P, Plemons J, Meyle J. Non–plaque-induced gingival diseases. Journal of Clinical Periodontology. 2018;**45**:S28-S43

[43] Li X, Zhang J, Zhang H, Li T. Biopsied non-dental plaque-induced gingival diseases in a Chinese population: A single-institute retrospective study. BMC Oral Health. 2021;**21**:1-8

[44] Clerehugh V, Tugnait A. Diagnosis and management of periodontal diseases in children and adolescents. Periodontology 2000. 2000;**2001**(26):146-168

[45] Clerehugh V, Tugnait A, Chapple ILC. Periodontal Management of Children, Adolescents and Young Adults. London: Quintessence Publishing Co. Ltd; 2004

[46] Clerehugh V. Periodontal diseases in children and adolescents. British Dental Journal. 2008;**204**:469-471

[47] Drummond BK, Brosnan MG, Leichter JW. Management of periodontal health in children: pediatric dentistry and periodontology interface. Periodontology 2000. Jun 2017;**74**(1):158-167

[48] Ainamo J, Nordblad A, Kallio P. Use of the CPITN in populations under 20 years of age. International Dental Journal. 1984;**34**:285-291

[49] Listgarten MA. Normal development, structure, physiology and repair of gingival epithelium. Oral Sciences Reviews. 1972;**1**:3-67

[50] Listgarten MA. Periodontal probing: What does it mean? Journal of Clinical Periodontology. 1980;**7**:165-176

[51] Van Der Velden U, De Vries JH. Introduction of a new periodontal probe: The pressure probe. Journal of Clinical Periodontology. 1978;**5**:188-197

[52] Goodson JM, Tanner ACR, Haffajee AD, Sornberger GC, Socransky SS. Patterns of progression and regression of advanced destructive periodontal disease. Journal of Clinical Periodontology. 1982;**9**:472-481

[53] Theil EM, Heaney TG. The validity of periodontal probing as a method of measuring loss of attachment. Journal of Clinical Periodontology. 1991;**18**:648-653

[54] Perry DA, Taggart EJ, Leung A. Comparison of a conventional probe with electronic and manual pressure regulated probes. Journal of Periodontology. 1994;**65**:908-913

[55] Clerehugh V, Kindelan S. Guidelines for periodontal screening and management of children and adolescents under 18 years of age. British Society of Periodontology and Implant Dentistry and British Society of Paediatric Dentistry. 2012;**1**:1-25

Section 3

Innovative Treatment Approaches

Chapter 5

Adjuvant Effect of Probiotics in the Treatment of Periodontal and Peri-Implant Diseases

Giovanni Barbagallo, Gianluca Monaca, Federica Di Gregorio, Gloria Alì, Vanina Porto and Giovanni Assenza

Abstract

Probiotics are "live microorganisms that can provide health benefits to the host when ingested in sufficient quantities". This category of microorganisms includes bacteria and yeasts that are normally present in the human intestine (intestinal microbiota) or similar to them. The introduction of beneficial microorganisms can modulate dysbiotic microbiota, restoring the normal host-microbiota balance. This creates the basis for the use of probiotics as adjunctive treatment in various pathologies such as metabolic diseases, tumors, neurological diseases, and inflammatory bowel diseases. The oral microbiota is a complex and diverse assembly of microorganisms that usually exist in balance with the host. An imbalance in it leads to the development of pathologies, including dental caries and periodontitis. The non-surgical treatment of choice for periodontitis aims at removing hard and soft deposits and disrupting the bacterial biofilm, although periodontal pockets can be immediately recolonized by pathogenic bacteria. The limitations of this therapeutic approach have led to the need for effective adjunctive treatments and support. Studies have shown that adding probiotics as adjuncts in the treatment of periodontitis and peri-implantitis reduces disease indices in both conditions.

Keywords: periodontitis, probiotics, dysbiosis, eubiosis, microbiome

1. Introduction

Probiotics are "live microorganisms that can provide health benefits to the host if ingested in sufficient quantities" [1–3]. This category of microorganisms includes bacteria and yeasts that are normally present in the human intestine (gut microbiota) or microorganisms similar to them. Probiotics include lactic acid bacteria (LAB), specifically Lactobacillus and Bifidobacterium, but also Enterococcus, Streptococcus, and Lactococcus. This category of microorganisms also includes *Escherichia coli* and Propionibacterium, which are less commonly used due to their potential adverse effects [4]. Probiotics are typically found in various food products, including yogurt, cheese, and other fermented products [5, 6]. Numerous studies have highlighted the beneficial effects of these microorganisms in treating various diseases [6].

IntechOpen

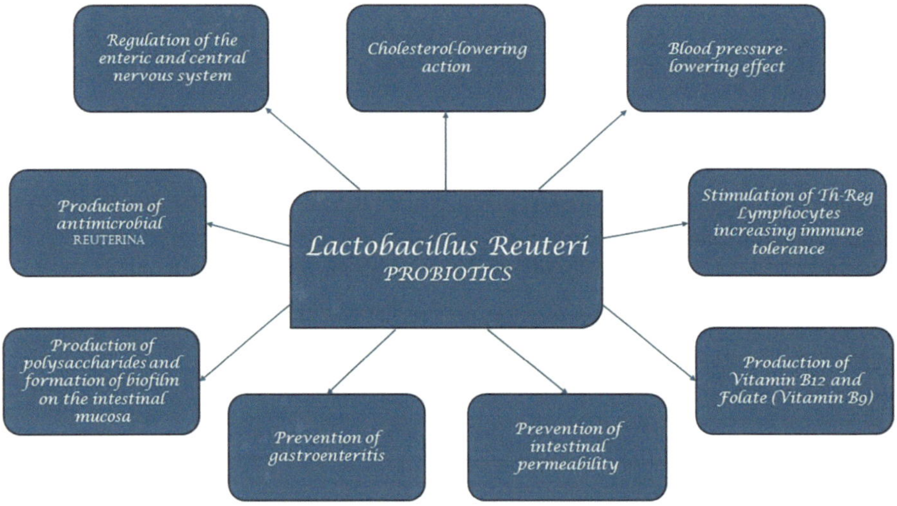

Figure 1.
Effect of Lactobacillus Reuteri.

Under normal conditions, humans are colonized by a variety of microorganisms. Healthy individuals usually have distinct and diverse microbial populations [6]. When the balance between microbiota and host is disrupted, dysbiosis occurs, leading to changes in microbial populations both qualitatively and especially quantitatively [7].

Studies have demonstrated a double relationship between the microbiota and the individual's health status. Among the various parts of the human body colonized by microorganisms, the gut is currently the most studied. Recent advances in genome sequencing, molecular techniques, and bioinformatics have highlighted a close association between gut microbiota, host health, and disease. Indeed, alterations in gut microbiota can cause disease, just as the persistence of certain diseases can lead to dysbiosis [6, 7]. Recent studies on the microbiota of the digestive system have shown similarities between the oral cavity microbiota and the gut microbiota; the latter also appears to be connected to the oral cavity microbiota (mouth-gut axis) [8]. Given the strong link between host health and microbiota, introducing beneficial microorganisms through the administration of probiotics can modulate dysbiotic microbiota, restoring the normal host-microbiota balance.

Figure 1 highlights some of the systemic benefits that can be obtained from the administration of probiotics; specifically, this image outlines the beneficial effects of L. reuteri on the human body.

2. Effects of probiotics as therapy in systemic pathologies

2.1 Metabolic diseases

The term metabolic disorders refer to a set of diseases characterized by variations and changes in the normal metabolic processes of the body.

In particular, obesity is a medical condition characterized by reduced activity of certain enzymes, which play a key role and are essential in lipid and carbohydrate metabolism, such as acetyl-coenzyme A (CoA) carboxylase and pyruvate dehydrogenase. This not only impairs the absorption and use of glucose by the body's cells but also increases the accumulation of lipids in both the liver and adipose tissue, thereby predisposing to the development of insulin resistance and type 2 diabetes [9].

Diabetes, a chronic disease characterized by elevated blood glucose levels, is also associated with dysregulation of several enzymes involved in carbohydrate and lipid metabolism. A study by Czumaj et al. highlighted the possible correlation between disorders of glucose absorption and utilization and abnormalities in the activity of enzymes such as glucokinase and hexokinase in diabetic subjects [9].

Multiple studies have highlighted the ability of probiotics to reduce inflammatory reactions, oxidative stress, and increase the length of adhesion proteins in the gastrointestinal epithelium. This results in a reduction of gut permeability, leading to improved insulin sensitivity and a reduced immune response [10].

Designer probiotics that express factors capable of influencing signals derived from adipose tissue, such as leptin, show potential therapeutic effects against these metabolic disorders [11]. They can influence hunger and eating behavior through the release of hormonal mediators (e.g., GLP-1 and peptide YY) that induce satiety. The effect of these hormones is a decrease in caloric intake through reduced hunger and increased satiety. Probiotics can also lower lipid absorption levels by breaking down triglycerides into glycerol and fatty acids, which are then eliminated in the intestine. The effects of probiotics on obesity have been analyzed in numerous randomized and controlled studies. These studies have shown that, compared to placebo, the use of probiotic supplements leads to a significant reduction in waist circumference, body weight, and body mass index. Quantitatively, the effects range from modest changes in some studies to substantial effects in others. Most studies have used Lactobacillus and Bifidobacterium, alone or in combination with other strains. Additional randomized studies have shown that the use of probiotics has improved the lipid profile, including reducing triglycerides, total cholesterol, and HDL cholesterol. Improvements in inflammatory levels (reduction of C-reactive protein and IL-6) and insulin sensitivity have also been reported with probiotic intake [6].

Phenylketonuria (PKU) is a hereditary disease characterized by a deficiency of the enzyme phenylalanine hydroxylase (PAH), leading to an increase in L-phenylalanine (Phe) levels in the blood. The treatment for PKU involves reducing Phe levels. Studies have demonstrated the effectiveness of engineered probiotics in reducing phenylalanine levels. Specifically, the use of genetically modified L. reuteri to provide phenylalanine lyase (PAL) has reduced Phe levels in the blood in mouse models of PKU [12]. Probiotics capable of expressing PAL and L-amino acid deaminase, which can break down Phe, are currently being studied in mouse models [13].

2.2 Cancer

The currently employed anti-tumor therapies are nonspecific treatments often incapable of achieving complete remission from tumors, and they frequently induce various side effects. In recent times, many patients are displaying increased resistance to these therapies.

Anaerobic bacteria capable of thriving in solid tumors could be harnessed for the delivery of anti-tumor agents and polysaccharides for the synthesis of nanodrugs [14]. In some studies, genetically modified probiotic bacteria have been created to express the viral thymidine kinase of Herpes Simplex. This recombinant bacterium has shown promising results in anti-tumor treatment [15, 16].

Bioengineered probiotics could be utilized to reduce chemotherapy-induced oral mucositis (OM) in oncology patients. L. lactis expressing human trefoil factor 1 administered in animal models has resulted in a reduction in OM [17].

2.3 Neurological diseases

Neurological disorders (ND) are diseases of the central nervous system characterized by the progressive loss of nervous tissue. The inability of neurons to regenerate after severe damage is what leads to the onset of these diseases. Currently, therapies for ND are solely aimed at managing the symptoms caused by these conditions. In-depth studies on some therapeutic agents currently used for the treatment of ND have shown the effectiveness of these drugs in controlling symptoms only in the short term. Moreover, these molecules cause significant side effects, including cognitive effects, hallucinations, impulse control disorders, confusion, urinary retention, and constipation [18].

Recently, a relationship has been demonstrated between the gut microbiome and abnormalities related to the central nervous system, including ND. Studies on animal models and clinical trials have highlighted a link between gut microbiota and abnormal behaviors, including depression. Further investigations conducted on subjects with depression found a return to normalcy of the gut microbiota after treatment with antidepressants [19].

Alzheimer's disease is a neurological disorder characterized by the accumulation of toxic proteins such as beta-amyloid (Aβ) plaques and tau. The drugs used to treat this condition, such as donepezil, belong to the family of cholinesterase inhibitors. Specifically, this drug presents various side effects, including gastrointestinal disorders, fatigue, and muscle cramps. In general, the efficacy of these drugs is still debated, and the response rate varies among different subjects. Additionally, about a third of patients discontinue the drug due to adverse effects [18].

Recent studies have analyzed the potential efficacy of probiotics, specifically L. plantarum, in improving learning and memory. This probiotic works by increasing the levels of acetylcholine, an essential neurotransmitter for memory and learning processing, and reducing those of acetylcholinesterase [20]. Studies administering 10^10 CFU of probiotics to animals (Bifidobacterium infantis, Lactobacillus fermentum, *L. acidophilus*, L. reuteri, B. longum, B. lactis, L. rhamnosus, and Lactobacillus reuteri) have shown that these probiotics may influence the production of superoxide dismutase (SOD), an important antioxidant, and inflammatory cytokines [18, 21].

Parkinson's disease (PD) is a neurological disorder characterized by the presence of motor and non-motor symptoms. Patients with this condition exhibit aggregation of alpha-synuclein (α-syn) into protofibrils, believed to be the toxic species mediating neuronal death by acting on various intracellular targets. It is believed that gastrointestinal inflammation increases the likelihood of neuroinflammation. Gastrointestinal pathogens also seem to be responsible for increasing motor symptoms and α-syn deposition [18].

The drug of choice for these patients is levodopa; despite its efficacy, levodopa has several side effects, and some symptoms, such as postural instability, show resistance to the drug [18]. Probiotics can influence the microbiome through antagonistic activities and by competing with pathogenic bacteria. These mechanisms could be important in patients with *H. pylori*, as this microorganism can lead to reduced levodopa absorption [22].

Studies conducted on Bifidobacterium breve, *Lactobacillus acidophilus*, L. brevis, B. infantis, and L. delbrueckii subsp. Bulgaricus, Streptococcus thermophilus, L. plantarum, B. longum, and L. paracasei have shown their ability to act on PPAγ, brain-derived neurotrophic factor, cell survival, and proliferation, which could lead to a reduction in inflammation [23]. Administration for 84 days of probiotics, including Bifidobacterium bifidum, Lactobacillus fermentum, *L. acidophilus*, and L. reuteri, has resulted in positive effects on the MDS-UPDRS (Movement Disorders Society-Unified Parkinson's Disease Rating Scale) [18].

Schizophrenia is a neurodegenerative disease that presents common symptoms such as delusions and hallucinations. Other symptoms include disorganized speech, cognitive, and negative symptoms. This pathology is characterized by dysfunction of neurotransmitters such as dopamine, glutamate, serotonin, norepinephrine, and GABA, leading to cognitive deficits [18].

The beneficial results obtainable through probiotic administration in subjects with schizophrenia may be due to anti-inflammatory effects, modulation of neurotransmitter levels, production of neurotrophic factors, and antioxidant activity. The use of Lactobacillus rhamnosus and Bifidobacterium lactis Bb12 leads to increased levels of BDNF, a neurotrophin associated with memory and learning ability, which is found in reduced quantities in subjects with schizophrenia [18]. Administration together with vitamin D associated with B. bifidum and lactobacilli seems to improve results obtained on the positive and negative syndrome scale (a rating scale used in medical fields to assess the severity of symptoms in subjects with schizophrenia) [24]. The evaluation of in vivo and clinical studies has demonstrated the efficacy of probiotics in reducing symptoms. Consequently, these microorganisms have the potential to mitigate the side effects caused by antipsychotics. Therefore, the use of probiotics in conjunction with standard therapy should be considered to reduce drug-related side effects, improve quality of life, and potentially alleviate psychotic symptoms [18].

2.4 Inflammatory bowel diseases

Inflammatory bowel diseases (IBD) are a group of diseases characterized by chronic and recurrent inflammation of the gastrointestinal tract. Of these pathologies, the most common are Crohn's disease (CD) and ulcerative colitis (UC). The exact etiology of IBD is still unknown, although alteration of the immune response toward the intestinal microbiota has been hypothesized as a possible cause. It is still unclear whether the dysfunctions leading to inflammation are related to a loss of immune tolerance toward a normal microbiota or to a normal immune response toward a dysbiotic microbiota [25].

Probiotics can counteract intestinal inflammatory processes by positively rebalancing the microbial environment and intestinal barrier permeability, improving the degradation of enteric antigens and altering their immunogenicity [25].

Studies conducted on Lactobacillus reuteri, administered to IL-10 knockout mice, have shown a preventive effect on the onset of colitis by increasing the number of lactobacilli in the gastrointestinal tract [26].

Analyses conducted on L. salivarius administered orally to IL-10 knockout mice have shown reduced inflammatory activity of the mucosa and reduced prevalence of colon cancer compared to mice treated with placebo. The results are due to the significant reduction in C. perfringens, coliforms, and enterococci [27].

3. Oral microbiome

The oral microbiota is a complex and diverse assemblage of microorganisms that typically exists in balance with the host [28]. It is the second largest in terms of composition and species variability (bacteria, archaea, protozoa, fungi, and viruses) after the gut microbiota. The colonization of the oral cavity begins just a few hours after birth, primarily by Staphylococcus epidermidis and some streptococci, particularly Streptococcus salivarius. A mature oral microbiome consists of about 700 species. The six major bacterial phyla are Firmicutes, Bacteroidetes, Proteobacteria, Actinobacteria, Spirochetes, and Fusobacteria [29, 30].

The mouth is similar to other body habitats in that it hosts a characteristic microbial community that provides benefits to the host. These microorganisms colonize the mucosal and dental surfaces of the mouth, forming structurally organized, multispecies, three-dimensional communities called biofilms (also known as "plaque") [31]. The microorganisms present in the biofilm are embedded in a matrix composed of polysaccharides they produce, as well as sugars, proteins, lipids, cellular fragments, and nucleic acids [32, 33].

In general, epithelial desquamation ensures that the microbial load on mucosal surfaces is kept relatively low. In contrast, the oral cavity is the only site in the body with non-desquamating surfaces that favor microbial colonization. This leads to the accumulation of a large number of microorganisms, particularly in stagnant and hard-to-reach areas, unless patients can maintain effective oral hygiene.

Many environmental factors influence the distribution and metabolic activity of the resident oral microbiota [34]. The mouth maintains a temperature of about 35–37°C, suitable for the growth of a wide range of microbes. The temperature increases in subgingival sites during inflammation, which can alter bacterial gene expression, modifying their competitiveness within the microbial community and promoting the growth and protease activity of specific pathogens. Although the oral cavity is a rich oxygen environment, facultative or obligate anaerobic bacteria predominate. The localization of these anaerobes in the oral cavity is usually related to the redox potential, a measure of the oxidative-reduction state of a particular site. The gingival sulcus, in healthy conditions, has the lowest Eh in the mouth and hosts the highest number of obligate anaerobes [35].

During the formation of the dental biofilm, the surface exposed to the environment is covered with a thin protein film to which colonizers adhere through various mechanisms. The first to adhere are gram-positive facultative anaerobes, defined as "early" colonizers, as they form a scaffold on which "late" microorganisms settle [29]. The bacteria of the subgingival plaque are primarily Corynebacterium, Streptococcus, Porphyromonas, Haemophilus/Aggregatibacter, Neisseriaceae, Fusobacterium, Leptotrichia, Capnocytophaga, and Actinomyces. These bacteria have a radial organization, "hedgehog-like": Corynebacterium produces filaments that form a supporting structure on which the other bacteria are orderly distributed, each in its position, with Streptococcus at the extremities creating a "corncob" configuration [29, 36, 37].

Saliva is rich in cellular aggregates of microorganisms from various oral surfaces, sometimes also associated with desquamated epithelial cells [38]. Saliva also contains secretory IgA and some antimicrobial peptides with defensive functions against infections. Saliva transports microorganisms from the oral cavity to the stomach and intestines, where the environment is more hostile, regulating their colonization [36]. The oral microbiome acts through "colonization resistance"; some bacteria can generate hydrogen peroxide and capture salivary amylase, initiating the digestive process of starch [36]. Another function is the conversion of nitrates to nitrites by some bacteria; nitrites are then converted to nitric oxide, involved in maintaining the tone of veins and arteries. Despite the positive functions performed by these microorganisms, their aggregation could easily allow them to enter the dense vascular network of the oral cavity and cause systemic diseases [32, 36].

4. Dysbiosis in the oral cavity

An imbalance in the oral microbiota leads to the development of pathologies, with the most common being dental caries and periodontitis (chronic conditions that progress slowly) [39].

4.1 Dental caries

Dental caries is one of the most widespread chronic multifactorial diseases in the population. The main factors that can lead to the onset of caries are predisposing factors in the host, dietary intake of carbohydrates, and the presence of acidophilic and acidogenic microorganisms in the oral cavity. The carious process arises from the disruption of the normally stable balance of the oral microbiome.

Microorganisms that colonize the oral cavity can form plaque on the surface of teeth, which has the characteristics of a classic biofilm. Specifically, bacteria that cause the carious process produce propionic, acetic, formic, and lactic acid as byproducts of carbohydrate metabolism. This results in a pH drop below 5.5, leading to proteolysis of the dental structure and demineralization of the enamel [38].

Lactobacilli and Streptococcus mutans have long been considered as pathogenic agents related to the cariogenic process. Recently, molecular analyses have shown the presence of a pathogenic community that also includes fungi (e.g., *Candida albicans*) and non-streptococcal microorganisms (e.g., Scardovia spp., Bifidobacterium spp., and Actinomyces spp.).

Different dental sites may present a different microbial composition. Microorganisms can interact synergistically to form a cariogenic biofilm within which the community changes as caries progresses, from early onset to deeper lesions with dentin exposure [39].

4.2 Periodontitis

Different microbial communities grow by adhering to the root surface of dental elements. These microbial populations are more protected against oxygen and masticatory loads compared to communities on supragingival surfaces. Subgingival populations receive nourishment primarily from crevicular fluid, an exudate with a composition similar to blood serum; this fluid flows into the sulcus from the adjacent gingival tissues. These populations are also partially nourished by salivary or dietary nutrients. Subgingival populations consist of viruses, bacteria, fungi, and archaea [40].

In subgingival plaque, the most abundant component is bacteria, with over 700 species. In individual subgingival sites, only a few bacterial species are numerically dominant. Studies on bacterial composition have identified Actinomyces naeslundii as the most frequently present subgingival species in a state of health.

Other Actinomyces spp., such as A. meyeri and A. odontolyticus, also appear in large numbers in healthy communities. Oral Actinomyces are gram-positive bacilli and are among the first microorganisms to colonize uncontaminated dental surfaces. They have the ability to organize with other early colonizing bacteria, such as Streptococcus, forming the scaffold of early dental plaque [41].

Numerous studies have highlighted significant qualitative differences in microbial composition between healthy sites and sites affected by periodontitis and peri-implantitis. In healthy sites, there is a higher abundance of Proteobacteria, including Clostridiales, Bradyrhizobiaceae, Alcaligenaceae, Burkholderiaceae, Lautropia, Escherichia, and Klebsiella, which are present specifically and almost exclusively [42].

In pathological sites, Mogibacterium, Dialister, Prevotella, Filifactor, Alloprevotella, and Olsenella are predominantly found. Recent studies show that Filifactor and Mogibacterium are associated with what was previously defined as "aggressive" periodontitis [43]. These species exhibit specific properties important in the pathogenic process of periodontal disease. Among the various microorganisms, Prevotella can stimulate periodontal inflammatory mechanisms through a Th17-mediated immune response, leading to neutrophil recruitment [44]. Filifactor, on the other hand, can stimulate the production of pro-inflammatory mediators capable of inducing the apoptotic process of gingival cells and causing a chronic inflammatory state [44, 45].

Bacterial species associated with health are also present in periodontitis, albeit in different percentages. This reinforces the principle that dysbiosis results from changes in dominant species rather than the de novo colonization of taxa associated with periodontitis [46].

Numerous factors contribute to the onset of dysbiosis. Undisturbed microbial accumulation in the gingival sulcus and the triggering of host responses lead to an increase in the outflow of gingival crevicular fluid from the tissues adjacent to the sulcus. It has been shown that the flow rate of gingival crevicular fluid gradually increases from health to gingivitis to periodontitis [47]. The enrichment of protease-rich bacterial communities, normally associated with periodontal disease, is favored by crevicular fluid [48]. Oxygen can also influence the microbiological structure. Bacterial families associated with gingivitis and health have greater resistance to oxygen compared to those associated with periodontal disease [49]. Tissue alteration and the presence of blood cell elements could also change subgingival populations, as some species, including black-pigmented anaerobic bacteria related to periodontal disease, prefer to use hemin derived from hemoglobin as an iron source.

It is necessary to emphasize the potential crucial role of certain bacterial species in orchestrating the development of dysbiosis. For example, P. gingivalis, a presumed significant pathobiont, can have a profound effect on the quantitative and qualitative composition of the commensal oral microbiome in periodontal disease. P. gingivalis induces dysbiosis in the normally benign oral microbiome, leading to the formation of a community structure responsible for tissue and bone destruction [50]. The mechanism by which P. gingivalis appears to act as an orchestrator of dysbiosis in model systems is likely related to mechanisms that disable and dysregulate the host's immune and inflammatory system, particularly the complement system [51]. Indeed, similar to other inflammatory pathologies, such as atherosclerosis, diabetes, and obesity, chronic stimulation triggers and induces the activation of the inflammasome, a multi-protein cytosolic complex involved in pathogen clearance and maintaining epithelial/mucosal barrier integrity. Further studies are still needed to confirm the involvement of the inflammasome in periodontal disease [52].

Environmental and behavioral factors, individual response, overall microbial load at the tooth-gingiva interface, type of microorganism, strains, and their interactions all contribute to predispose the individual to the initiation and progression of periodontitis. Through this complex network of interactions, a specific expression pattern can be determined that causes the transition from health to periodontitis. Key pathogenic microorganisms can play a decisive role in altering homeostasis and inducing dysbiosis in the subgingival biofilm [28, 53, 54].

Literature shows that no single microbial species is sufficient alone to cause periodontitis. For inflammatory bone loss to occur, the participation of key pathogens that subvert the host response by disrupting homeostasis and pathobionts that enhance the dysfunctional host response, leading to dysbiotic inflammation, is necessary. Dysbiosis does not depend on a specific microbial composition but on combinations of specific genes or the collective virulence of microorganisms within the dysbiotic microbial community [55].

Considering all this, the most promising strategies to inhibit this dysbiosis involve restoring homeostasis rather than controlling infection through antimicrobial agents. Conservative approaches to eubiotic species are those that can prevent or reverse the transition to a dysbiotic community.

Periodontal diseases, encompassing a range of alterations from gingivitis to periodontitis, are among the most common pathological processes in the oral cavity. Periodontitis is a chronic disease characterized by gingival inflammation and loss of connective attachment, leading to tooth loss due to alveolar bone resorption. About 50% of individuals over the age of 30 and over 60% of those over the age of 65 are affected by periodontitis. This pathological condition can arise when there is a loss of balance in the oral microbiome. The primary etiology of chronic periodontitis is represented by the microbial biofilm; however, this pathology can be modulated by many other systemic and local agents. The species Tannerella forsythia and Porphyromonas gingivalis are the most pathogenic. Nonetheless, Aggregatibacter actinomycetemcomitans is also among the species involved in the development of periodontitis.

So far, the modalities of treatment for periodontal disease have been classified as non-surgical and surgical procedures, sometimes completed with the administration of systemic antibiotics. The most commonly chosen treatment is scaling and root planing (SRP), in conjunction with oral hygiene instructions, due to its good results, although periodontal pockets can be immediately recolonized by pathogenic bacteria. The limitations of these treatments in the presence of sites with high probing depths and the resistance due to the overuse of antibiotics have compelled the search for alternative approaches that enhance the effects of SRP and have reduced adverse effects [56, 57].

Studies have shown that the chronic inflammatory state resulting from periodontitis influences various systemic diseases, such as cardiovascular diseases, diabetes, and respiratory disorders. Supporting this, a study by Monsarrat et al. [58] hypothesized a link between periodontitis and fifty-seven systemic diseases. This lays the foundation for considering common pathophysiological processes and guiding professionals toward evidence-based and patient-centered approaches for concomitant pathological conditions [58]. This is why its treatment is so important at a systemic level. In the treatment of chronic periodontitis, the primary goal is to address the primary etiology. Effective therapy results in the reduction of periodontal pocket depth with improvements in clinical attachment levels. Additional therapies, such as probiotics, can be useful in these multifactorial conditions where scaling and root planing alone have not succeeded, as they provide benefits against caries and in the periodontal field, clinical, microbiological, and inflammatory improvements are observed [56, 57].

Probiotics are defined by the World Health Organization as live cultures of microorganisms that provide a health benefit to the host when taken in sufficient quantities. The idea that probiotic microorganisms can influence health status originates with bacteriologist Metchnikoff, who observed that life expectancy in Bulgaria was higher. He hypothesized that this was due to a higher intake of fermented milk, which has a high content of L. bulgaricus. Studies on probiotics have shown beneficial effects in various systemic alterations, including urogenital diseases and gastrointestinal disorders. To be defined as probiotics, microorganisms must be resistant to bile acids, able to adhere to and colonize the intestinal mucosa, and be safe in animals. Currently, their role in modulating periodontal diseases is not fully understood [57].

4.3 Peri-implant diseases

Dental implants are dental devices representing a therapeutic strategy for both replacing a missing tooth due to caries, periodontal disease, trauma, or agenesis, and restoring entire dental arches. The advent of implantology has enabled many patients destined for prosthetic therapy with removable devices to receive fixed prosthetic treatments. Over the last forty years, there has been extensive use of these devices linked to their effectiveness and the belief that implants, once osseointegrated, were a definitive treatment; however, over time, this conviction has been abandoned following the occurrence of various technical and biological complications [59].

Among the biological complications that can affect dental implants, two different clinical conditions can be distinguished: peri-implant mucositis and peri-implantitis. Both are inflammatory pathologies affect the tissues around dental implants. The triggering etiological factor for these conditions is the peri-implant biofilm [60].

Peri-implant mucositis is characterized by inflammation of the mucosa around the implant without marginal bone resorption; clinically, bleeding on probing is observed. Mucositis is a reversible condition that, if left untreated, can progress to peri-implantitis [60, 61].

Peri-implantitis is a pathological process causing inflammation of the peri-implant mucosa and progressive bone resorption. Clinically, increased probing depth and/or recession of the mucosal margin, inflammation, suppuration, and/or bleeding on probing are observed; there is also evidence of bone resorption compared to previous radiographic evaluations [60, 61]. Among the main risk factors, it is important to consider poor oral hygiene, a history of severe previous periodontitis, and poor adherence to peri-implant support therapy (PIST) after implant placement. There is less evidence in the literature regarding smoking, diabetes, or implant placement that limits access to oral hygiene and maintenance [60].

The pathophysiological mechanism underlying peri-implant diseases is comparable to the mechanism that characterizes periodontal diseases. In fact, it is possible to identify analogies between the pathophysiological mechanism of peri-implant mucositis and biofilm-induced gingivitis and between peri-implantitis and periodontitis. However, there are anatomical differences between the tissues surrounding the tooth and those surrounding the implant that influence the onset and progression of these diseases. Unlike periodontal tissues, peri-implant tissues lack cementum and periodontal ligament; therefore, around the dental implant, there are only two layers: alveolar bone and peri-implant mucosa. The mucosa also presents differences: the peri-implant epithelial attachment is usually longer, the connective tissue does not have fibers inserted in the supracrestal area, and vascularization is reduced [60]. The peri-implant biofilm is the main etiological factor of peri-implant diseases.

The peri-implant biofilm is a complex multispecies community above and below the mucosa that develops following exposure to the oral cavity [62]. The dental implant, being inserted into the oral cavity, is exposed to the microorganisms that make up the oral microbiome. Indeed, since they are in the same environment, the dental and peri-implant biofilms have similar characteristics [63]. A study comparing the microbiological composition of biofilms in peri-implant and adjacent periodontal sites highlighted a similarity in the microbiological composition of the biofilm between the sites. Higher levels of T. forsythia, P. micra, *F. nucleatum*, Fusobacterium necrophorum, and C. rectus were found in peri-implant samples compared to periodontal samples. In peri-implant sites with high inflammatory indices, a higher percentage of T.denticola, *P. intermedia*, Staphylococcus warnery, and *P. intermedia* were found compared to healthy sites. Additionally, the microbiota of smokers showed greater diversity compared to healthy non-smokers or those with pathology [64]. The similarity between the peri-implant microbiota and the periodontal microbiota has been found in both health and disease (periodontitis and peri-implantitis). The microbiota associated with peri-implant mucositis appears to be similar to that associated with peri-implantitis [65, 66].

5. The microbiology of periodontitis and peri-implantitis

Under physiological conditions, the oral cavity is populated by more than 700 bacterial species, which colonize not only the tooth surface but also surrounding structures such as the oral epithelium, hard and soft palate, and the dorsal surface of the tongue. It is essential, therefore, to select potential probiotic bacterial strains in such a way as to ensure the absence of pathogenic genetic sequences, which could be deleterious to the oral bacterial community and, consequently, oral health. In this regard, a list of safe probiotic microorganisms for humans has been compiled for introduction into foods. This list includes a series of strains of lactobacilli and streptococci [56].

5.1 Antibacterial activity against periodontopathic bacteria

Numerous strains of lactobacilli and streptococci, observed in healthy oral cavities, exhibit antibacterial activity against Porphyromonas gingivalis, *Prevotella intermedia*, Aggregatibacter actinomycetemcomitans, and *Fusobacterium nucleatum*. The inhibitory activity of certain Lactobacillus species against multiple microbial species has been demonstrated through various studies. For example, Lactobacillus fermentum is active against microaerophiles, while Lactobacillus gaseri is active against anaerobes. Other strains of Lactobacillus, including Lactobacillus paracasei and *Lactobacillus acidophilus*, hinder the growth and proliferation of Staphylococcus aureus, a pathogen present in more severe forms of periodontitis. Streptococci also inhibit anaerobic bacteria, such as P. gingivalis and *P. intermedia*, through the synthesis of lactic acid and other organic acids. Some probiotic strains isolated in yogurt-based commercial products produce hydrogen peroxide, through which they inhibit P. gingivalis. One study demonstrated that the STYM1 strain of Lactobacillus delbrueckii releases intracellular proteins capable of stimulating the synthesis of inhibitory concentrations of hydrogen peroxide. Hydrogen peroxide can be produced and generated by various enzymes in many strains of Lactobacillus, including pyruvate oxidase, lactate oxidase, NADH oxidase, and NADH flavin-dependent reductase. In one study, the growth of P. gingivalis in agar plates treated with hydrogen peroxide from L. delbrueckii hydrogenase was significantly inhibited compared to untreated plates [56].

5.2 Antibacterial effects mediated by bacteriocins

The term bacteriocin was first used in the 1950s by Francois Jacob. They are proteins or peptides of bacterial origin that are extremely stable and resistant, produced indiscriminately by both gram-positive and gram-negative bacteria, with inhibitory activity against bacterial strains different from the producing strain, but phylogenetically related to it. Several studies have highlighted how bacteriocins are a valuable system among the possible defense mechanisms employed by bacteria, contributing significantly to the antibacterial activity of many probiotics, including lactobacilli. They exhibit peculiar characteristics, synthesized at the ribosomal level, and they have a limited spectrum of action with bactericidal activity exerted only against bacteria closely related to the producing strain and are effective at nanomolar concentrations. They are classified into three main classes based on their molecular sizes and functions. Among the bacteriocins relevant for the oral cavity are included salivaricin from Lactobacillus salivarius and Streptococcus salivarius, reuterin from Lactobacillus reuteri, plantaricin from Lactobacillus plantarum, and nisin from Lactobacillus lactis. Plantaricin contributes to the improvement of systemic health and, in the context of oral health, prevents the growth of P. gingivalis. Salivaricin eliminates bacteria associated with halitosis, while reuterin has potential applications for periodontal disease, as it shows antibacterial effects against Tannerella forsythia ATCC 43037. Similarly, nisin has antibacterial action against multiple gram-negative periodontal pathogens including P. gingivalis, *P. intermedia*, A. actinomycetemcomitans, *F. nucleatum*, and Treponema denticola, in addition to its effects on gram-positive bacteria associated with the gastrointestinal tract. Finally, nisin has no cytotoxic effects in humans, specifically at the level of the various cells lining the oral cavity or relevant to the periodontium [56].

5.3 Beneficial colonizing properties

Probiotics have a shorter assimilation time within the oral cavity compared to other parts of the digestive system. It is ideal for oral probiotics to have a high colonizing potential, which includes the ability to adhere to oral epithelial cells. Unlike the intestine, the oral epithelial tissue is composed of a thin mucosa coated with mucin, which, due to its viscosity, allows microbes to attach directly to the oral epithelium. Some strains of streptococcus, including *S. sanguinis* and S. salivarius, exhibit strong colonizing properties due to the presence on their surface of filamentous accessory structures, called pili, formed by pilins and adhesins, which help bacteria adhere to mucin. Within minutes of probiotic intake, various strains of streptococcus, such as *S. sanguinis*, S. gordonii, S. oralis, and S. mitis, quickly attach to the salivary biofilm covering the tooth surface, connecting to it through receptors. In some simulated tests on human teeth, it has been observed that lactobacilli usually have a lower adherence capacity compared to streptococci when it comes to hydroxyapatite coated with saliva.

In the oral environment, lactobacilli and bifidobacteria compete with the pathogen P. gingivalis in terms of adherence. These probiotics alter the interaction of epithelial cells with P. gingivalis by modulating its ability to adhere to and invade these cells [56].

5.4 Mechanisms of action of probiotics

The mechanisms of action of probiotics are not always well understood; therefore, they are mainly documented through in vitro studies or animal models. The mode of action may be related to the modulation of the host's microbiota.

- One widely recognized mode of action is the barrier effect or "resistance to colonization" exerted against pathogenic bacteria, which prevents or limits their colonization. Inhibition can be caused by the production of broad-spectrum bacteriocins, by metabolites such as short-chain fatty acids, which cause a decrease in pH, unfavorable to bacterial growth, or by biosurfactants with antimicrobial activity. Other ways in which the barrier effect manifests include competition for binding sites and inhibition of adhesion [67].

- A second mode of action involves enhancing the barrier function of the intestinal mucosa, related to the quality of tight junctions between intestinal epithelial cells. Probiotics can operate at the level of signaling pathways, leading to increased mucus layer or defensin production, and on tight junction proteins.

- Finally, a third mode involves modulation of the immune system. Some structural elements repeated on the surface of microorganisms recognize specific receptors on innate immune cells (pattern recognition receptors, PRRs) and trigger the activation of regulatory T lymphocytes and the differentiation of T-helper lymphocytes, thereby inducing the formation of pro- or anti-inflammatory cytokines. Bacteria with probiotic potential can have different effects depending on the profile of stimulated cytokines [68, 69].

5.5 The dosage and administration method of probiotics

The mode of administration of probiotics is solely oral. There are various preparations available on the market in the form of capsules, tablets, powders, yogurt, or other functional foods. The authors recommend oral administration through tablets to dissolve in the mouth, as the probiotic has greater retention in the oral cavity, thus allowing for more extensive colonization of various available niches. Probiotics in various oral intake modalities must have a high concentration of the chosen bacterium; only then, by overcoming the gastric barrier, can they colonize further parts of the digestive tract. In **Figure 2**, some probiotics available on the market are shown.

It has been observed that the efficacy of probiotics, administered for 3 months (90 days), remains for a maximum duration of 6 months (180 days), beyond which a new administration cycle should begin [70]. The authors recommend taking one probiotic tablet to dissolve in the mouth once a day on an empty stomach for 30 days and then discontinuing for an additional 3 months, at the end of which another cycle can be started.

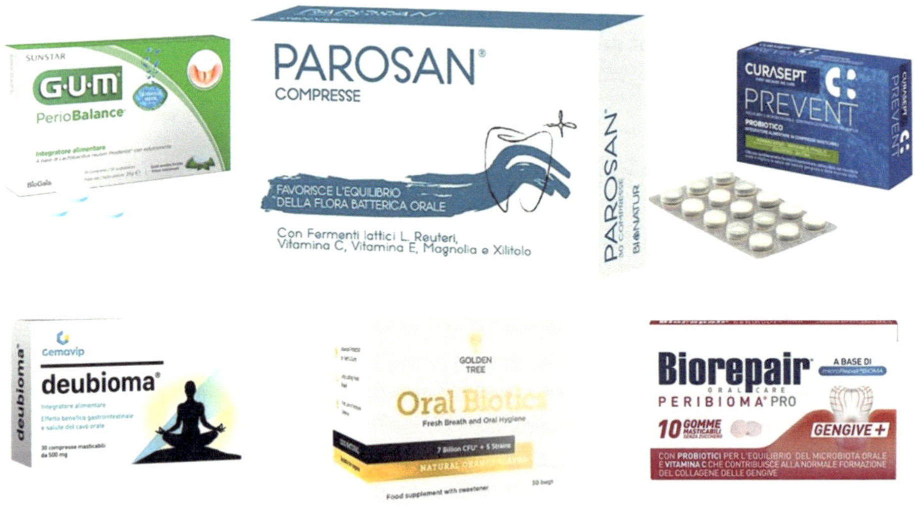

Figure 2.
Some probiotics available on the market.

6. Non-surgical periodontal therapy (NSPT)

In the literature, different endpoints have been evaluated to establish the effectiveness of treatment phases, often considering more frequently the mean reduction in pocket probing depth (PPD) and the increase in clinical attachment level (CAL). It is therefore indispensable to define more appropriate endpoints to achieve after periodontal therapy. For example, in the guidelines of the European Federation of Periodontology (EFP), a precise definition of the desired outcome after the treatment of stage I-III periodontitis has been established. Upon completion of periodontal therapy, a patient is defined as stable if they exhibit stable periodontal health with reduced periodontium (bleeding on probing in a total of sites less than 10%; probing depth equal to or less than 4 mm and no sites of 4 mm with bleeding on probing). After completing non-surgical periodontal treatment, if these criteria are met but bleeding on probing is present in more than 10% of sites, the patient is diagnosed with stable periodontitis with gingival inflammation. Sites with bleeding on probing and maintaining a probing depth > 4 mm require additional therapy as they are likely unstable sites. It should be kept in mind that individuals who have successfully treated and stabilized periodontal disease still maintain the risk of recurrence; in these individuals, if bleeding on probing is present, interventions are necessary to reduce inflammation and prevent disease progression. If the objectives are not achieved with this sequence of steps 1 and 2 (removal of supragingival dental biofilm, patient lifestyle change, and control and elimination of subgingival biofilm and tartar), it is necessary to proceed to step 3 of periodontal treatment, which consists of various subgingival instrumentation and/or surgical approaches. After completing phase 3, it is necessary to evaluate the results obtained; if the predefined objectives are achieved, rigorous periodic maintenance therapy is still indispensable [71, 72].

The acronym non-surgical periodontal therapy (NSPT) indicates the second phase of periodontal treatment, based on subgingival mechanical instrumentation.

Normally, NSPT is performed through root planning and scaling (SRP); this type of treatment is considered the best for managing stage I-III periodontitis. However, in some patients and/or sites, this type of treatment does not produce sufficient results. This poor response may be due to the persistence of an inflammatory response or the treatment's inability to restore a state of eubiosis due to the persistence of subgingival biofilm in the pocket [71].

In light of this, there is ongoing research into additional therapies that can improve the results of subgingival instrumentation alone. Regarding the use of probiotics as adjuncts to periodontal therapy, a recent study analyzed the adjunct effects of these supplements on microbiological, immunological, and clinical outcomes after NSPT. Ten randomized studies were considered, where all subjects underwent NSPT; subsequently, some received probiotics or a placebo as an adjunct, while others received neither. Probiotic intake led to significant results at 3 and 12 months, resulting in a reduction in PPD at 12 months. In pockets with probing depth ≥ 5 mm, probiotics showed significant results in reducing CAL and probing depth. At 3 months, no significant difference was found between the groups in pathogen levels [71].

Similarly, Matsubara et al. [73] in a literature review concluded that oral administration of probiotics is a safe and effective addition to conventional mechanical treatment (SRP) in managing periodontitis and that their additional use improves disease indices and reduces the need for further antibiotics [73]. Also, Vives-Soler et al. [74] through a systematic literature review evaluated the efficacy of various probiotic strains as adjuncts to non-surgical periodontal therapy, establishing that probiotics can provide additional benefit to mechanical debridement [74]. Supporting this, a study conducted by Monaca et al. [75], involving the intake of a probiotic tablet in the oral cavity until complete dissolution without chewing or swallowing it, showed a statistically significant improvement in probing depth in patients with peri-implantitis for the first six months; while regarding patients with periodontal disease, sites with probing depth between 4 and 6 mm showed a statistically significant improvement. Sites with a probing depth exceeding 6 mm gained clinical attachment; however, some remained above values associated with the risk of recurrence: consequently, they were subsequently treated surgically [75].

7. Treatment of peri-implant diseases

Biological complications affecting implants are currently a topic of high interest in the field of dentistry as there is still no validated therapeutic procedure. Peri-implant mucositis is a reversible condition; hence, treating this condition results in resolving it and restoring peri-implant health. If left untreated, it may lead to the onset of peri-implantitis, which can cause the loss of the affected implant and consequently the prosthesis supported by the implant [60].

The treatment of peri-implant mucositis aims to reduce inflammation of the soft tissues by removing hard and soft deposits from the surface of the dental implant and the overlying prosthetic structure without scratching the abutment or implant collar surface. Removal can be performed using ultrasound, curettes, rotating or oscillating brushes. The desired outcome is the elimination of inflammation, clinically detectable by the absence of bleeding on probing and suppuration. If treatment goals are not achieved within three months, it is advisable to repeat the treatment. If the prosthesis supported by the implant does not allow adequate home or professional cleansing, removal or modification of the prosthesis is necessary [60]. In cases of mucositis, the use of local antibiotics is not recommended, while the administration of chlorhexidine or probiotics as adjuncts to mechanical therapy may be considered for a limited time [60].

The treatment of peri-implantitis aims to halt bone resorption by addressing the bacterial insult that causes tissue damage. This is achievable through reducing the pathogenic bacterial flora in peri-implant pockets, tissue conditioning, and decontamination of the implant surface. In cases where sites are difficult to maintain with home and professional hygiene procedures, corrective and/or site reduction procedures are necessary. Additionally, it is crucial to enroll the patient in a strict support program. Whenever possible, bone defect reconstruction is recommended [76]. Currently, there is no strongly validated therapy; treatment of peri-implantitis is based on approaches already widely validated for the treatment of periodontitis. Treatment consists of non-surgical and surgical phases. The main goal of non-surgical therapy is to reduce inflammation by removing peri-implant biofilm. Therapy involves supra- and sub-gingival mechanical decontamination using ultrasonic instruments or curettes. This treatment does not show significant results, and in most cases, a surgical approach is necessary [60].

The surgical approach aims to gain access to the implant to decontaminate normally inaccessible surfaces and create a positive anatomy of peri-implant hard and soft tissues. Whenever possible, bone defect reconstruction is necessary [77]. Surgical procedures include reconstructive surgery, open-flap debridement (OFD), and resective surgery (apically positioned flap, APF).

Open-flap debridement is a surgical procedure that, by elevating a flap, reduces microbial load at the implant area using a mechanical approach. The use of a flap allows access to areas unreachable with non-surgical procedures [78]. Indeed, studies have shown that OFD results in greater decontamination of implant surfaces compared to non-surgical treatment and may promote new osseointegration, especially on rough implant surfaces [65].

Resective surgery is a technique indicated for non-esthetic peri-implant defects. The technique involves a phase of osteoplasty and/or ostectomy and a phase of decontamination and possible polishing of the exposed implant surface, after which the flap is repositioned apically. Resective surgery has limited long-term efficacy and is indicated only for shallow bone defects in non-esthetic areas where reconstructive procedures are not recommended [79].

Reconstructive surgery is a surgical procedure that aims, in addition to mechanical decontamination of surfaces, to reconstruct the bone defect. The technique involves elevating a flap to access the defect, decontaminating the implant surface, and finally using biomaterials (bone grafts, membranes, amelogenins, or other bioactive agents) to reconstruct the defect [60]. Given the absence of a protocol for peri-implantitis treatment that determines stable long-term results, there is a need to seek adjuncts that can improve therapy outcomes. Probiotics may play a modulating and protective role against pathogenic bacterial colonization and promote a microbiota capable of supporting peri-implant health [80]. Currently, there is limited evidence in the literature regarding the efficacy of probiotics as adjuncts to peri-implant disease treatment. Studies on L. reuteri have shown improvement in clinical parameters and pro-inflammatory cytokines in implants affected by mucositis [80, 81] and peri-implantitis [75, 80].

8. Conclusions

Significant interindividual variability of the human microbiome mediated by factors such as age, diet, antibiotic use, dietary supplements, underlying medical conditions, and circadian activity patterns can influence the effects of probiotics. Regarding their activity on periodontal diseases, it is mandatory to evaluate how the effects vary depending on the means of probiotic microorganism administration and its ability to colonize the oral cavity; furthermore, its therapeutic benefits need to be assessed, as well as its survival in the oral cavity.

In conclusion, although further studies are needed to evaluate the modes of application, different therapeutic regimens, and the persistence of probiotic microorganisms in the oral cavity after discontinuation of probiotic therapy, there is ample evidence supporting the use of probiotics with promising results that promote their possible use as an adjunctive treatment to non-surgical periodontal therapy [71, 75].

Conflict of interest

The authors declare no conflict of interest.

Author details

Giovanni Barbagallo[1,2]*, Gianluca Monaca[1,2], Federica Di Gregorio[1,2], Gloria Alì[1,2], Vanina Porto[2,3] and Giovanni Assenza[1,2]

1 DDS, DMD, Italy

2 Centro Odontoiatrico Mediterraneo in Agreement with NHS, Private Dental Practice, Catania, Sicily, Italy

3 BDH, MSAT, Italy

*Address all correspondence to: giobar1201@gmail.com

References

[1] Mailander-Sanchez D, Wagener J, Schaller M. Potential role of probiotic bacteria in the treatment and prevention of localised candidosis. Mycoses. 2012;**55**(1):17-26

[2] Silva DR, Sardi JDCO, Pitangui NDS, Roque SM, Silva ACBD, Rosalen PL. Probiotics as an alternative antimicrobial therapy: Current reality and future directions. Journal of Functional Foods. 2020;**73**:104080

[3] Hill C, Guarner F, Reid G, Gibson GR, Merenstein DJ, Pot B, et al. Expert consensus document: The international scientific association for probiotics and prebiotics consensus statement on the scope and appropriate use of the term probiotic. Nature Reviews. Gastroenterology & Hepatology. 2014;**11**:506-514

[4] Boyle RJ, Robins-Browne RM, Tang ML. Probiotic use inclinical practice: What are the risks. The American Journal of Clinical Nutrition. 2006;**83**(6):1256-1264

[5] Zheng BD, Gan L, Tian LY, Chen GH. Protein/polysaccharide-based hydrogels loaded probiotic-mediated therapeutic systems: A review. International Journal of Biological Macromolecules. 2023;**253**(Pt 2):126841

[6] Debnath N, Yadav P, Mehta PK, Gupta P, Kumar D, Kumar A, et al. Designer probiotics: Opening the new horizon in diagnosis and prevention of human diseases. Biotechnology and Bioengineering. 2024;**121**(1):100-117

[7] Al-Rashidi HE. Gut microbiota and immunity relevance in eubiosis and dysbiosis. Saudi Journal of Biological Sciences. 2022;**29**(3):1628-1643

[8] Kitamoto S, Kamada N. The oral-gut axis: A missing piece in the IBD puzzle. Inflammation and Regeneration. 2023;**43**(1):54. DOI: 10.1186/s41232-023-00304-3. PMID: 37932859; PMCID: PMC10626704

[9] Czumaj A, Szrok-Jurga S, Hebanowska A, Turyn J, Swierczynski J, Sledzinski T, et al. The pathophysiological role of CoA. International Journal of Molecular Sciences. 2020;**21**:9057

[10] Gomes AC, Bueno AA, de Souza RGM, Mota JF. Gut microbiota, probiotics and diabetes. Nutrition Journal. 2014;**13**:60. DOI: 10.1186/1475-2891-13-60

[11] Chen Z, Guo L, Zhang Y, Walzem RL, Pendergast JS, Printz RL, et al. Incorporation of therapeutically modified bacteria into gut microbiota inhibits obesity. Journal of Clinical Investigation. 2014;**124**(8):3391-3406

[12] Durrer KE, Allen MS, Hunt von Herbing I. Genetically engineered probiotic for the treatment of phenylketonuria (PKU); assessment of a novel treatment in vitro and in the PAHenu2 mouse model of PKU. PLoS One. 2017;**12**(5):e0176286

[13] Isabella VM, Ha BN, Castillo MJ, Lubkowicz DJ, Rowe SE, Millet YA, et al. Development of a synthetic live bacterial therapeutic for the human metabolic disease phenylketonuria. Nature Biotechnology. 2018;**36**(9):857-864

[14] Taniguchi S, Fujimori M, Sasaki T, Tsutsui H, Shimatani Y, Seki K, et al. Targeting solid tumors with non-pathogenic obligate anaerobic bacteria. Cancer Science. 2010;**101**(9):1925-1932

[15] Wang C, Ma Y, Hu Q, Xie T, Wu J, Zeng F, et al. Bifidobacterial recombinant thymidine kinase-ganciclovir gene therapy system induces FasL and TNFR2 mediated antitumor apoptosis in solid tumors. BMC Cancer. 2016;**16**(1):545

[16] Zhou H, He Z, Wang C, Xie T, Liu L, Liu C, et al. Intravenous administration is an effective and safe route for cancer gene therapy using the Bifidobacterium-mediated recombinant HSV-1 thymidine kinase and ganciclovir. International Journal of Molecular Sciences. 2016;**17**(6):891

[17] Caluwaerts S, Vandenbroucke K, Steidler L, Neirynck S, Vanhoenacker P, Corveleyn S, et al. AG013, a mouth rinse formulation of Lactococcus lactis secreting human trefoil factor 1, provides a safe and efficacious therapeutic tool for treating oral mucositis. Oral Oncology. 2010;**46**(7):564-570

[18] Aghamohammad S, Hafezi A, Rohani M. Probiotics as functional foods: How probiotics can alleviate the symptoms of neurological disabilities. Biomedicine & Pharmacotherapy. 2023;**163**:114816

[19] Shen Y, Yang X, Li G, Gao J, Liang Y. The change of gut microbiota in MDD patients under SSRIs treatment. Scientific Reports. 2021;**11**(1):14918

[20] Nimgampalle M, Kuna Y. Anti-Alzheimer properties of probiotic, lactobacillus plantarum MTCC 1325 in Alzheimer's disease induced albino rats. Journal of Clinical and Diagnostic Research: JCDR. 2017;**11**(8):KC01

[21] Mehrabadi S, Sadr SS. Assessment of probiotics mixture on memory function, inflammation markers, and oxidative stress in an Alzheimer's disease model of rats. Iranian Biomedical Journal. 2020;**24**(4):220

[22] Gazerani P. Probiotics for Parkinson's disease. International Journal of Molecular Sciences. 2019;**20**(17):4121

[23] Tan AH, Hor JW, Chong CW, Lim SY. Probiotics for Parkinson's disease: Current evidence and future directions. JGH Open. 2021;**5**(4):414-419

[24] Szeligowski T, Yun AL, Lennox BR, Burnet PW. The gut microbiome and schizophrenia: The current state of the field and clinical applications. Frontiers in Psychiatry. 2020;**11**:156

[25] Cabezas-Cruz A, Bermúdez-Humarán LG. Exploring the relationship between Faecalibacterium duncaniae and *Escherichia coli* in inflammatory bowel disease (IBD): Insights and implications. Computational and Structural Biotechnology Journal. 2023;**19**(23):1-9

[26] Madsen KL, Doyle JS, Jewell LD, Tavernini MM, Fedorak RN. Lactobacillus species prevents colitis in interleukin 10 gene-deficient mice. Gastroenterology. 1999;**116**(5):1107-1114

[27] O'Mahony L, Feeney M, O'Halloran S, Murphy L, Kiely B, Fitzgibbon J, et al. Probiotic impact on microbial flora, inflammation and tumour development in IL-10 knockout mice. Alimentary Pharmacology & Therapeutics. 2001;**15**(8):1219-1225

[28] Nibali L, Henderson B. The human microbiota and chronic disease: Dysbiosis as a cause of human pathology. Wiley Blackwell. 2016. DOI: 10.1002/9781118982907

[29] Kriebel K, Hieke C, Müller-Hilke B, Nakata M, Kreikemeyer B. Oral biofilms from symbiotic to pathogenic interactions and associated disease -connection of periodontitis and rheumatic arthritis by Peptidylarginine deiminase. Frontiers in Microbiology.

2018;**30**(9):53. DOI: 10.3389/fmicb.2018.00053. PMID: 29441048; PMCID: PMC5797574

[30] Dewhirst FE, Chen T, Izard J, Paster BJ, Tanner AC, Yu WH, et al. The human oral microbiome. Journal of Bacteriology. 2010;**192**(19):5002-5017. DOI: 10.1128/JB.00542-10. Epub 2010 Jul 23. PMID: 20656903; PMCID: PMC2944498

[31] Simon-Soro A, Ren Z, Krom BP, Hoogenkamp MA, Cabello-Yeves PJ, Daniel SG, et al. Polymicrobial aggregates in human saliva build the Oral biofilm. MBio. 2022;**13**(1):e0013122. DOI: 10.1128/mbio.00131-22. Epub 2022 Feb 22. PMID: 35189700; PMCID: PMC8903893

[32] Mosaddad SA, Tahmasebi E, Yazdanian A, Rezvani MB, Seifalian A, Yazdanian M, et al. Oral microbial biofilms: An update. European Journal of Clinical Microbiology & Infectious Diseases. 2019;**38**(11):2005-2019. DOI: 10.1007/s10096-019-03641-9. Epub 2019 Aug 1. PMID: 31372904

[33] Li X, Liu Y, Yang X, Li C, Song Z. The Oral microbiota: Community composition, influencing factors, pathogenesis, and interventions. Frontiers in Microbiology. 2022;**29**(13):895537. DOI: 10.3389/fmicb.2022.895537. PMID: 35572634; PMCID: PMC9100676

[34] Marsh PD, Moter A, Devine DA. Dental plaque biofilms: communities, conflict and control. Periodontology 2000. 2000;**55**(1):16-35. DOI: 10.1111/j.1600-0757.2009.00339.x. PMID: 21134226

[35] Kenney EB, Ash MM Jr. Oxidation reduction potential of developing plaque, periodontal pockets and gingival sulci. Journal of Periodontology. 1969;**40**(11):630-633. DOI: 10.1902/jop.1969.40.11.630. PMID: 5260618

[36] Tuganbaev T, Yoshida K, Honda K. The effects of oral microbiota on health. Science. 2022;**376**(6596):934-936. DOI: 10.1126/science.abn1890. Epub 2022 May 26. PMID: 35617380

[37] Mark Welch JL, Rossetti BJ, Rieken CW, Dewhirst FE, Borisy GG. Biogeography of a human oral microbiome at the micron scale. Proceedings of the National Academy of Sciences of the United States of America. 2016;**113**(6):E791-E800. DOI: 10.1073/pnas.1522149113. Epub 2016 Jan 25. PMID: 26811460; PMCID: PMC4760785

[38] Struzycka I. The oral microbiome in dental caries. Polish Journal of Microbiology. 2014;**63**(2):127-135. PMID: 25115106

[39] Lamont RJ, Koo H, Hajishengallis G. The oral microbiota: Dynamic communities and host interactions. Nature Reviews. Microbiology. 2018;**16**(12):745-759. DOI: 10.1038/s41579-018-0089-x. PMID: 30301974; PMCID: PMC6278837

[40] Moore WE, Moore LV. The bacteria of periodontal diseases. Periodontology 2000. 1994;**5**:66-77. DOI: 10.1111/j.1600-0757.1994.tb00019.x. PMID: 9673163

[41] Diaz PI, Chalmers NI, Rickard AH, Kong C, Milburn CL, Palmer RJ Jr, et al. Molecular characterization of subject-specific oral microflora during initial colonization of enamel. Applied and Environmental Microbiology. 2006;**72**(4):2837-2848. DOI: 10.1128/AEM.72.4.2837-2848.2006. PMID: 16597990; PMCID: PMC1449052

[42] Barbagallo G, Santagati M, Guni A, Torrisi P, Spitale A, Stefani S, et al. Microbiome differences in periodontal,

peri-implant, and healthy sites: A cross-sectional pilot study. Clinical Oral Investigations. 2022;**26**(3):2771-2781. DOI: 10.1007/s00784-021-04253-4. Epub 2021 Nov 26. PMID: 34826030

[43] Nibali L, Sousa V, Davrandi M, Spratt D, Alyahya Q, Dopico J, et al. Differences in the periodontal microbiome of successfully treated and persistent aggressive periodontitis. Journal of Clinical Periodontology. 2020;**47**(8):980-990. DOI: 10.1111/jcpe.13330. Epub 2020 Jun 26. PMID: 32557763

[44] Fine DH, Markowitz K, Fairlie K, Tischio-Bereski D, Ferrendiz J, Furgang D, et al. A consortium of Aggregatibacter actinomycetemcomitans, streptococcus parasanguinis, and Filifactor alocis is present in sites prior to bone loss in a longitudinal study of localized aggressive periodontitis. Journal of Clinical Microbiology. 2013 Sep;**51**(9):2850-2861. DOI: 10.1128/JCM.00729-13. Epub 2013 Jun 19. PMID: 23784124; PMCID: PMC3754677

[45] Moffatt CE, Whitmore SE, Griffen AL, Leys EJ, Lamont RJ. Filifactor alocis interactions with gingival epithelial cells. Molecular Oral Microbiology. 2011;**26**(6):365-373. DOI: 10.1111/j.2041-1014.2011.00624.x. Epub 2011 Sep 13. PMID: 22053964; PMCID: PMC3248241

[46] Abusleme L, Dupuy AK, Dutzan N, Silva N, Burleson JA, Strausbaugh LD, et al. The subgingival microbiome in health and periodontitis and its relationship with community biomass and inflammation. The ISME Journal. 2013;7(5):1016-1025. DOI: 10.1038/ismej.2012.174. Epub 2013 Jan 10. PMID: 23303375; PMCID: PMC3635234

[47] Hatipoğlu H, Yamalik N, Berberoğlu A, Eratalay K. Impact of the distinct sampling area on volumetric features of gingival crevicular fluid. Journal of Periodontology. 2007;**78**(4):705-715. DOI: 10.1902/jop.2007.060331. PMID: 17397319

[48] ter Steeg PF, Van der Hoeven JS, de Jong MH, van Munster PJ, Jansen MJ. Enrichment of subgingival microflora on human serum leading to accumulation of Bacteroides species, Peptostreptococci and Fusobacteria. Antonie Van Leeuwenhoek. 1987;**53**(4):261-272. DOI: 10.1007/BF00393933. PMID: 3674857

[49] Diaz PI, Zilm PS, Rogers AH. *Fusobacterium nucleatum* supports the growth of Porphyromonas gingivalis in oxygenated and carbon-dioxide-depleted environments. Microbiology (Reading). 2002;**148**(Pt 2):467-472. DOI: 10.1099/00221287-148-2-467. PMID: 11832510

[50] Darveau RP, Hajishengallis G, Curtis MA. Porphyromonas gingivalis as a potential community activist for disease. Journal of Dental Research. 2012;**91**(9):816-820. DOI: 10.1177/0022034512453589. Epub 2012 Jul 6. PMID: 22772362; PMCID: PMC3420389

[51] Hajishengallis G, Liang S, Payne MA, Hashim A, Jotwani R, Eskan MA, et al. Low-abundance biofilm species orchestrates inflammatory periodontal disease through the commensal microbiota and complement. Cell Host & Microbe. 2011;**10**(5):497-506. DOI: 10.1016/j.chom.2011.10.006. Epub 2011 Oct 27. PMID: 22036469; PMCID: PMC3221781

[52] Marchesan JT, Girnary MS, Moss K, Monaghan ET, Egnatz GJ, Jiao Y, et al. Role of inflammasomes in the pathogenesis of periodontal disease and therapeutics. Periodontology

2000. 2020;**82**(1):93-114. DOI: 10.1111/prd.12269. PMID: 31850638; PMCID: PMC6927484

[53] Kornman KS. Mapping the pathogenesis of periodontitis: A new look. Journal of Periodontology. 2008;**79**(8 Suppl):1560-1568. DOI: 10.1902/jop.2008.080213. PMID: 18673011

[54] Berglundh T, Liljenberg B, Lindhe J. Some cytokine profiles of T-helper cells in lesions of advanced periodontitis. Journal of Clinical Periodontology. 2002;**29**(8):705-709. DOI: 10.1034/j.1600-051x.2002.290807.x. PMID: 12390567

[55] Lamont RJ, Hajishengallis G. Polymicrobial synergy and dysbiosis in inflammatory disease. Trends in Molecular Medicine. 2015;**21**(3):172-183. DOI: 10.1016/j.molmed.2014.11.004. Epub 2014 Nov 20. PMID: 25498392; PMCID: PMC4352384

[56] Nguyen T, Brody H, Radaic A, Kapila Y. Probiotics for periodontal health-current molecular findings. Periodontology 2000. 2021;**87**(1):254-267. DOI: 10.1111/prd.12382. PMID: 34463979; PMCID: PMC8448672

[57] Canut-Delgado N, Giovannoni M, Chimenos-Küstner E. Are probiotics a possible treatment of periodontitis? Probiotics against periodontal disease: A systematic review. British Dental Journal. 2021;**231**(10):1-7. DOI: 10.1038/s41415-021-3624-5

[58] Monsarrat P, Blaizot A, Kémoun P, Ravaud P, Nabet C, Sixou M, et al. Clinical research activity in periodontal medicine: A systematic mapping of trial registers. Journal of Clinical Periodontology. 2016;**43**:390-400. DOI: 10.1111/jcpe.12534

[59] Carassi A, Cortellini P, Trombelli L. Parodontologia e Terapia Implantare, Quintessenza Edizioni, Milano. 2016. 6a edizione, 2 volumi

[60] Herrera D, Berglundh T, Schwarz F, Chapple I, Jepsen S, Sculean A, et al. EFP workshop participants and methodological consultant. Prevention and treatment of peri-implant diseases-the EFP S3 level clinical practice guideline. Journal of Clinical Periodontology. 2023;**50**(Suppl. 26):4-76. DOI: 10.1111/jcpe.13823. Epub 2023 Jun 4. PMID: 37271498

[61] Berglundh T, Armitage G, Araujo MG, Avila-Ortiz G, Blanco J, Camargo PM, et al. Peri-implant diseases and conditions: Consensus report of workgroup 4 of the 2017 world workshop on the classification of periodontal and Peri-implant diseases and conditions. Journal of Periodontology. 2018;**89** (Suppl. 1):S313-S318. DOI: 10.1002/JPER.17-0739. PMID: 29926955

[62] Quirynen M, Zhao H, Soers C, Dekeyser C, Pauwels M, Coucke W, et al. The impact of periodontal therapy and the adjunctive effect of antiseptics on breath odor-related outcome variables: A double-blind randomized study. Journal of Periodontology. 2005;**76**(5):705-712. DOI: 10.1902/jop.2005.76.5.705. PMID: 15898930

[63] Lang NP, Berglundh T. Working group 4 of seventh European workshop on periodontology. Periimplant diseases: Where are we now?--consensus of the seventh European workshop on periodontology. Journal of Clinical Periodontology. 2011;**38**(Suppl. 11): 178-181. DOI: 10.1111/j.1600-051X.2010.01674.x. PMID: 21323713

[64] Sahrmann P, Gilli F, Wiedemeier DB, Attin T, Schmidlin PR, Karygianni L. The microbiome of peri-implantitis:

A systematic review and meta-analysis. Microorganisms. 2020;**8**(5):661. DOI: 10.3390/microorganisms8050661. PMID: 32369987; PMCID: PMC7284896

[65] Máximo MB, de Mendonça AC, Renata Santos V, Figueiredo LC, Feres M, Duarte PM. Short-term clinical and microbiological evaluations of peri-implant diseases before and after mechanical anti-infective therapies. Clinical Oral Implants Research. 2009;**20**(1):99-108. DOI: 10.1111/j.1600-0501.2008.01618.x. PMID: 19126114

[66] Casado PL, Otazu IB, Balduino A, de Mello W, Barboza EP, Duarte ME. Identification of periodontal pathogens in healthy periimplant sites. Implant Dentistry. 2011;**20**(3):226-235. DOI: 10.1097/ID.0b013e3182199348. PMID: 21613949

[67] Gupta V, Garg R. Probiotics. Indian Journal of Medical Microbiology. 2009;**27**(3):202-209. DOI: 10.4103/0255-0857.53201. PMID: 19584499

[68] Round JL, Mazmanian SK. The gut microbiota shapes intestinal immune responses during health and disease. Nature Reviews. Immunology. 2009;**9**(5):313-323

[69] Ménard O, Butel MJ, Gaboriau-Routhiau V, WaligoraDupriet AJ. Gnotobiotic mouse immune response induced by Bifidobacterium sp. strains isolated from infants. Applied and Environmental Microbiology. 2008;**74**(3):660-666

[70] Pelekos G, Ho SN, Acharya A, Leung WK, McGrath C. A double-blind, paralleled-arm, placebo-controlled and randomized clinical trial of the effectiveness of probiotics as an adjunct in periodontal care. Journal of Clinical Periodontology. 2019;**46**(12):1217-1227. DOI: 10.1111/jcpe.13191. Epub 2019 Oct 28. PMID: 31479530

[71] Haas AN, Furlaneto F, Gaio EJ, Gomes SC, Palioto DB, Castilho RM, et al. New tendencies in non-surgical periodontal therapy. Brazilian Oral Research. 2021;**35**(Suppl. 2):e095. DOI: 10.1590/1807-3107bor-2021.vol35.0095. PMID: 34586209

[72] Sanz M, Herrera D, Kebschull M, Chapple I, Jepsen S, Beglundh T, et al. Treatment of stage I-III periodontitis-the EFP S3 level clinical practice guideline. Journal of Clinical Periodontology. 2020;**47**(S22 Suppl. 22):4-60. DOI: 10.1111/jcpe.13290

[73] Matsubara VH, Bandara HMHN, Ishikawa KH, Mayer MPA, Samaranayake LP. Il ruolo dei batteri probiotici nella gestione della malattia parodontale: una revisione sistematica. Expert Review of Anti-Infective Therapy. 2016;**14**(7):643-655. DOI: 10.1080/14787210.2016.1194198

[74] Vives-Soler A, Chimenos-Küstner E. Effect of probiotics as a complement to non-surgical periodontal therapy in chronic periodontitis: A systematic review. Medicina Oral, Patología Oral y Cirugía Bucal. 2020;**25**(2):e161-e167. DOI: 10.4317/medoral.23147. PMID: 31893476; PMCID: PMC7103449

[75] Monaca G, Di Gregorio F, Alì G, Russo P, Barbagallo G. Effetto Adiuvante dei probiotici nel trattamento della malattia parodontale e perimplantare. Il Dentista Moderno, Giugno. 2023;**6**:70-76

[76] Mombelli A. Microbiology and antimicrobial therapy of peri-implantitis. Periodontology 2000. 2002;**28**:177-189. DOI: 10.1034/j.1600-0757.2002.280107.x. PMID: 12013341

[77] Renvert S, Polyzois I, Maguire R. Re-osseointegration on previously contaminated surfaces: A systematic

review. Clinical Oral Implants Research. 2009;**20**(Suppl. 4):216-227. DOI: 10.1111/j.1600-0501.2009.01786.x. PMID: 19663967

[78] Heitz-Mayfield LJA, Salvi GE, Mombelli A, Faddy M, Lang NP. Anti-infective surgical therapy of peri-implantitis. A 12-month prospective clinical study. Clinical Oral Implants Research. 2012;**23**(2):205-210. DOI: 10.1111/j.1600-0501.2011.02276.x. Epub 2011 Aug 9. PMID: 22092831

[79] Khoury F, Keeve PL, Ramanauskaite A, Schwarz F, Koo KT, Sculean A, et al. Surgical treatment of peri-implantitis - consensus report of working group 4. International Dental Journal. 2019;**69**(Suppl. 2):18-22

[80] Galofré M, Palao D, Vicario M, Nart J, Violant D. Clinical and microbiological evaluation of the effect of lactobacillus reuteri in the treatment of mucositis and peri-implantitis: A triple-blind randomized clinical trial. Journal of Periodontal Research. 2018;**53**(3):378-390. DOI: 10.1111/jre.12523. Epub 2018 Jan 19. PMID: 29352461

[81] Flichy-Fernández AJ, Ata-Ali J, Alegre-Domingo T, Candel-Martí E, Ata-Ali F, Palacio JR, et al. The effect of orally administered probiotic lactobacillus reuteri-containing tablets in peri-implant mucositis: A double-blind randomized controlled trial. Journal of Periodontal Research. 2015;**50**(6):775-785. DOI: 10.1111/jre.12264. Epub 2015 Feb 25. PMID: 25712760

Chapter 6

Introduction to Diode Laser Therapies in Dentistry

Santiago Arias-Herrera, Rebeca Sánchez-Martos and Lourdes Alfaro-Ochoa

Abstract

Actually, there are different types of lasers that can be used in dentistry, being the diode laser one of the most popular. The therapies in which diode laser is used are photothermic therapy, which is subdivided into low- and high-intensity photothermal therapy and photodynamic therapy. Photothermic therapy is based on an increase in local temperature, allowing the incision, excision, ablation, and vaporisation of the tissues, as well as haemostasis and coagulation of lesions. It also produces bacterial decontamination through thermal photo disinfection. Low-intensity photothermic therapy also achieves an analgesic, anti-inflammatory, and healing effect. On the other hand, photodynamic therapy facilitates bacterial decontamination through activated photodisinfection in combination with a photoactive substance. These therapies can be used in a separate way or combined, obtaining different results depending on the tissue in which they are applied and according to the technical specifications used. Therefore, the diode laser, thanks to its versatility, applicability, and good clinical results in specialities such as endodontics, periodontics, surgery, or implantology, should be considered as an implement of transversal application in contemporary dentistry.

Keywords: dentistry, diode laser, photothermal therapy, photodynamic therapy, cellular biostimulation

1. Introduction

The application of laser in medicine is one of the most used and developed treatments in recent years. It was first introduced to the health field in dermatology in 1960 [1]. Laser technology is developing very rapidly, allowing for the diversification of lasers in the field of dentistry. The word LASER as it is commonly known today, comes from the initials of its acronym: "Light Amplification by Stimulated Emission of Radiation". The laser is an electro-optic device that, when stimulated, emits a beam of monochromatic light with high-intensity energy [2].

Dermatology was the first medical speciality to introduce laser therapy in 1995. That is when the clinical uses and limitations were presented. The main function with which it was presented was selective photothermolysis in common vascular and pigmented conditions of the skin and mucous membranes, including infants and children. The results were effective and quickly evaluated, being incorporated into the daily practice of the moment [1].

Lasers were introduced into the field of clinical dentistry with the hope of overcoming some of the drawbacks posed by conventional dental procedure methods [3]. Among the first studies such as that of Maiman et al. in 1960 [4] about the first operative laser, already introduced the use of the laser itself in the world of dentistry. The first laser studies on dental tissues, such as the one carried out by Stern and Sognnaes in 1965, already reported significant clinical effects on tooth structure *in vivo* and *in vitro* with the ruby laser. In these articles, the absence of heat harmful to oral tissues or sensitive dental pulp has already been demonstrated [5].

Nowadays, dental lasers are widely used in the dental field around the world, allowing patients to be provided with high-quality treatments in minimally invasive dentistry [6, 7].

1.1 Mechanism of action

A laser is a device that produces coherent electromagnetic radiation. Therefore, light amplification by stimulated emission of radiation, known as LASER for short, is an electro-optic device that produces a narrow and highly energised monochromatic beam of radiation of a specific wavelength. Depending on the wavelength of the laser and where it is applied, different optical phenomena may occur [8].

It is light, so it has the basic properties of optics, such as transmission, absorption, reflection, and refraction. The absorption by the tissues of the incident light energy on the irradiated tissues will be the one that releases their energy [2]. The emitting units of laser energy allow for the variation of some parameters related to the amount of energy released per unit of time, or what is the same, the power. The handpieces that will facilitate the transport of energy to the target tissue are usually provided with optics that will allow us, depending on the distance of application, to concentrate or distribute the laser energy on a smaller or larger application surface [9]. Thus, when we apply a certain amount of energy per unit of time, we obtain a higher power density on a small surface than when we apply it to a larger surface. Power density will determine different effects on the same tissue [10].

The emitting units of laser energy allow for the variation of some parameters related to the amount of energy released per unit of time, or what is the same, the power. The handpieces that will facilitate the transport of energy to the target tissue are usually provided with optics that will allow us, depending on the distance of application, to concentrate or distribute the laser energy on a smaller or larger application surface. Thus, when we apply a certain amount of energy per unit of time, we obtain a higher power density on a small surface than when we apply it to a larger surface. Power density will determine different effects on the same tissue [10, 11].

2. Laser in dentistry

2.1 Types of lasers most used in dentistry

Lasers in dentistry are diverse and, as mentioned above, will be specific according to the target tissue to be treated. That is why they will be divided into specialities to talk about the most used in each of the areas. Specifically in oral implantology and periodontology, they are the CO_2 laser, the diode laser, the Nd: YAG laser and the Er: YAG laser. These have, in this area, as main utility, debridement treatments, subgingival curettage (in scaling and root planing), and periodontal surgeries such as open flap, which are complementary to mechanical debridement. Other surgical procedures found with these lasers are bone recontouring, and implant maintenance, in prophylaxis of mucositis or peri-implantitis [12, 13]. Nd:YAG lasers have the advantage of being used whether or not they come into contact with the medium to be treated. Er: YAG lasers are mostly used in the decontamination of implant surfaces without causing any detrimental effect on the surrounding bone. In those treatments on teeth, it has been shown that CO2 lasers are safe for use on hydroxyapatite, the main dental component [14, 15].

2.1.1 CO_2 laser

The CO_2 laser belongs to the group of high-power lasers. Its medium is the gaseous state, and it has a wavelength of around 9600–10,600 nm. Its waveform is described as continuous superpulsed. Due to its characteristics, it is absorbed by soft tissues, producing temperature increases of around 1700°C in the target tissue. As an advantage, it presents less heating in the adjacent tissues with respect to other less surface-absorbed lasers [9, 16].

The main use of the CO_2 laser in dentistry is focused on the specialities of oral implantology and periodontics, as well as the diode laser, the Nd:YAG laser and the Er: YAG laser. Specifically for tissue cuts such as incision, soft tissue ablation, and gingival de-epithelialisation in periodontal regenerative procedures. In addition, in the treatment of dental implants for disinfection, bone recontouring, and the maintenance of implants, in the prophylaxis of mucositis or peri-implantitis [17].

2.1.2 Nd:YAG laser

The neodymium:yttrium-aluminium-garnet (Nd:YAG) laser belongs to the group of high-power lasers. Its medium is the solid state, and it has a wavelength of around 1064 nm. Its waveform is pulsed. As a disadvantage, studies point out that both the Nd:YAG laser and the diode laser present a risk of thermal accumulation in adjacent tissues, since they are not well absorbed by soft tissues. That is why they should not exceed 65°C to avoid necrosis of the same [9].

The use of the Nd:YAG laser in dentistry is focused on the specialities of oral implantology and periodontology, as well as the diode laser, the CO_2 laser and the Er: YAG laser. It is also used in dental therapy, specifically for tissue cuts such as incision, soft tissue ablation, haemostasis, periodontal decontamination, and in dental therapy for vaporisation of incipient caries, treatment of dentin hypersensitivity, and root canal decontamination in endodontics [9, 18].

2.1.3 Er: YAG laser

The Erbium, yttrium-aluminium-garnet (Er: YAG) laser's waveform is described as continuous pulsed. Its medium is the solid state, and it has a wavelength of around 2940 nm [10].

Among the main uses are tissue cuts such as incision, soft tissue ablation, haemostasis, periodontal decontamination, and in dental therapy for vaporisation of incipient caries, treatment of dentin hypersensitivity and root canal decontamination in endodontics. The biomechanical preparation of the root canal is carried out in a conventional way, but there are publications in which Er, Cr:YSGG or Er: YAG lasers are used for this purpose. Both the Er: YAG laser and the Er, Cr:YSGG laser have shown high disinfection in exposed dentin, where it is common to find smears with the presence of bacteria, that is, caries [8].

2.1.4 Diode laser

The diode laser corresponds like the previous ones, to high-power lasers. This type of laser is not visible, and the transmission is by fibre optics and infrared, continuous wave. It shows variations in its wavelength presentation, from 810 to 980 nm. Hence, it is versatile in its forms [19]. Depending on their power, diode lasers can be classified into two large groups. Low-power diode lasers are also called soft lasers due to their low energy. They emit in the region of the near-infrared or red spectrum (632.8, 670 and 830 nm wavelength), with an average power of 1–100 mW. Its main clinical applications are based on its biostimulatory effect and its analgesic-anti-inflammatory effect. The other type of diode laser is High Power. Lasers with powers between 1 and 15 W or higher and with a wavelength between 810 and 980 nm. In accordance with international classifications regarding the safety measures to be taken into account when using these devices, the European Union (ISO) and the United States (ANSI) regulations consider the diode laser a type IV laser [8, 9].

2.2 Laser therapies

In addition to the physical foundations of laser operation, the response of the tissues to laser light must also be taken into account. The oral cavity is a very complex application area for laser therapy [16]. This is due to the fact that it has highly differentiated and specialised areas. Hard and mineralised tissues such as teeth or bone tissue, as well as soft tissues. All these structures have different optical characteristics and will not respond in the same way to the same laser or the same wavelength [20].

Treatment guidelines, and therefore therapies, depend on the laser used and the thermal effects to be achieved on the target tissue. In order to advance in the understanding of laser therapy in oral tissues, it is necessary to understand, first, the main photobiological effects. These are the effects that the laser beam produces when it is absorbed by the oral tissues. The main photobiological effects are photothermal and photochemical effects [21]. The most widely used diode laser therapies are based on these two principles.

3. Photothermal diode laser therapy

Photothermic therapy was the first to be studied; lasers produce a thermal effect on tissues, which translates into very precise cuts, vaporisation, and coagulation of small blood vessels [16]. This therapy is based on the conversion of light energy into thermal energy, increasing the temperature in the tissues and producing injuries that will depend on the degrees reached [8, 20].

Photothermic therapy can be divided into two distinct varieties. High- and low-intensity photothermal therapy [22]. Although both employ the same principle of thermal energy, high-intensity therapy derives its benefits from increasing the temperature produced by the laser beam in the tissues, while low-intensity therapy focuses more on cellular biostimulation instead of temperature (**Table 1**).

Diode laser therapy		Mechanism of action	Biological effect
Photothermal laser therapy	High-intensity photothermal therapy	Thermal energy	Bemostatic cut Coagulation Bactericidal and bacteriostatic
	Low-intensity photothermal therapy	Photon-cell interaction	Cell biostimulation Analgesic Anti-inflammatory
Photodynamic therapy	Photochemical therapy	Photochemical reaction	Bactericidal and bacteriostatic

Table 1.
Summary of diode laser therapies.

3.1 High-intensity diode photothermal therapy

3.1.1 Mechanism of action

In order to perform high-intensity photothermal therapy, it is necessary to have a diode laser capable of emitting a wavelength between 810 and 980 nm and with powers between 1 and 15 W. The photothermal interaction is characterised by an increase in local temperature induced by the action of the laser [6, 7]. Thus, the main photothermal interactions are tissue incision/excision, ablation/vaporisation, and haemostasis/coagulation. The light energy contacts the tissue for a certain time (exposure time) and produces a thermal interaction [5–7, 18].

Depending on the temperature reached, the effect will vary. Bacterial inactivation occurs when the temperature reaches 37–50°C [21]. When the temperature rises to 60–70°C, protein coagulation and denaturation are observed [6, 7, 13]. If the temperature is 100°C, the histological water vaporisation occurs in a phenomenon called vaporysis, a process that results in tissue ablation [21]. In the event that the thermal process exceeds 200°C, an effect called carbonisation occurs, where the carbon develops as the final product of thermolysis and acts by dissipating heat, causing potential trauma to the adjacent tissues [16, 18].

3.1.2 Main indications

The first speciality in dentistry to implement the use of diode laser photothermal therapy was surgery, and today, it continues to be one of its main indications for use [8, 9]. When the use of the diode laser was implemented in this speciality there was already experience in the use of the CO2 laser; however, a less aggressive laser with soft tissues was necessary and one that was safe to use close to the teeth since the diode laser is less absorbed by the water of the mineralised tissue. The main advantage of the diode laser in surgery is its great haemostatic cutting effect, which makes it ideal when excision is intended, limiting bleeding [23]. However, the diode laser can be used to perform all types of soft tissue surgeries such as the removal of benign lesions. Especially indicated for soft tissue injuries near the teeth. In most cases, the lesions heal by the second intention, so there is no need for a suture [24]. We can successfully use the diode laser in the treatment of excision of a wide variety of benign tumours of the oral cavity, such as papillomas, ranulas, mucoceles, fibromas, focal epithelial hyperplasia of the oral cavity, recurrent aphthae, epulis, melanic spots, etc.

Therefore, the main advantages of diode laser in surgery are less postoperative swelling, improvement in tissue healing and reduction in scar formation [11, 23].

Another speciality in which diode laser photothermal therapy is widely used is periodontics. The main benefit sought with the application of lasers in periodontics is bacterial decontamination [25]. It is a great help in areas of difficult access where the benefit of conventional treatments is more limited, such as furcations or deep pockets [26]. One of the most used lasers in periodontics is Er: YAG, with its bactericidal effects against periodontopathogenic bacteria [27]; it also eliminates bacterial endotoxins and the temperature reached by the cement was kept within clinically safe limits for dental pulp [26, 27]. However, the root morphology obtained after instrumentation with the Er: YAG laser has been the subject of study, since it has been reported that the root surfaces treated with this laser show an irregular, chalky appearance with isolated craters, which could favour bacterial recolonisation [28]. The current lines of research are focused on the use of the diode laser since its bactericidal efficacy has been well documented [29]. Mainly in colonies of *Actinobacillus actinomycetemcomitans*, this bacterium is associated with the most aggressive forms of periodontal disease, and diode laser can be an aid where the classic treatment of scaling and root planing is less effective [16, 26].

Photothermic therapy with diode laser in implantology has been used mainly for the treatment of peri-implant pathologies [16, 18, 26]. The term "peri-implant diseases" collectively refers to the inflammatory processes that take place in the tissues surrounding an implant [30] and follow the same principles as in the speciality of periodontics, seeking its bactericidal effect and tissue biostimulation. The evidence obtained in experimental studies in animals and humans shows that the main etiological factor involved in the development of peri-implant pathologies is the accumulation of biofilm [31, 32]. However, despite the fact that the evidence in periodontal studies demonstrated the bactericidal effectiveness of the diode laser and its safety in periodontal and dental tissues, it was necessary to investigate its interaction with the titanium structure of dental implants to allow its use in implantology [16, 18]. This interaction is observed in a study carried out by Romanos et al. In 2000, they compared *in vitro* the effects of Nd:YAG and diode lasers (980 nm) on titanium discs that simulated dental implants. Their results were that, contrary to what happened with the Nd:YAG laser, the discs subjected to the diode laser were not damaged or modified [33]. Showing, therefore, that the diode laser does not change the surface of dental implants and that it can be used in the treatment of peri-implant diseases. Several studies have reported better results in the resolution of peri-implant pathologies by adding diode laser photothermal therapy to mechanical debridement [32]. This is due to its bactericidal effect against the main periodontopathogens together with its ability to biostimulate tissue in deep layers [33]. These characteristics allow the laser to act against the main etiological factor of peri-implant pathologies in addition to favouring the response of the tissues to the treatment [24]. However, although the results are promising, more research is needed to determine if photothermal diode laser therapy can alleviate the limitations of conventional therapy in the treatment of these pathologies [32, 34]. **Figure 1** shows the 300 μ optical fibre tip of the 890 nm diode laser being used in the treatment of peri-implant mucositis.

Similar to how it occurs in periodontics and implantology, the bactericidal effect of the diode laser can also be used in the endodontic treatment of teeth [34, 35]. One of the main objectives of endodontic treatment is to leave the root canal free of microorganisms [36]. For this, different disinfection systems can be used, and the diode laser is one of them. However, caution must be taken to prevent possible thermal damage generated by the laser on the periodontium or the tooth itself. Photothermal disinfection of root canals can increase root canal dentin

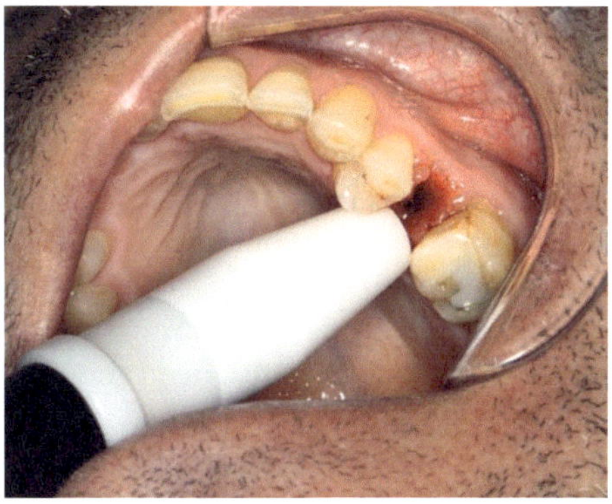

Figure 1.
Fox III diode laser (a.R.C. Laser GmbH, Nürnberg, Germany) 300 μ optical fibre tip being used in the treatment of peri-implant mucositis.

temperatures, but periodontal fluid circulation has a cooling effect on the outer root surface, reducing the risk of potential thermal injury to periodontal tissue [37]. Several studies have shown that this laser can be used with up to 4.5 W of power with an exposure time of 60 seconds, achieving a correct bacterial elimination from the canal (**Table 2**) [38].

3.1.3 Contraindications

The main contraindications of diode laser photothermal therapy derive from one of its main characteristics, which is the high penetration of the thermal action in deep layers [24]. This effective penetration of the laser is what allows biostimulation of oral soft tissues; however, it can be a disadvantage on certain occasions. For example, its use in the removal of premalignant or malignant lesions is more limited due to the high penetration capacity of the laser, which will cause an area of cellular biostimulation in deep tissue layers [9, 11]. This could lead to a recurrence of the lesion if it were not completely excised with wide margins of safety. For the treatment of these lesions, the use of the CO_2 laser is more indicated [10].

Another element to take into account, especially in surgery, is that its haemostatic effect is much lower compared to the CO_2 laser, so it will only be useful for excision of superficial lesions, and it will not be recommended for excision of angiomatous lesions or for surgical interventions in which profuse bleeding is expected [23].

The diode laser is also not indicated for taking biopsies [10]. Because the use of laser with a marked thermal effect can alter the structure of the margins of the lesion and make the anatomopathological analysis of the sample difficult, in these cases, it is more advisable to use a cold scalpel [24].

Oral Surgery	Periodontics	Implantology	Endodontics
• Remove benign oral lesions • Haemostatic cut	• Coadjuvant treatment of periodontal disease	• Coadjuvant treatment of peri-implant pathologies	• Root canal desinfection

Table 2.
Main indications in dentistry for high inesity photothermal therapy.

Regarding the use of diode laser in the treatment of periodontal diseases and peri-implant pathologies, although it can be used as an adjunctive treatment in the management of these pathologies, it should never be used as an alternative to mechanical debridement [20, 26]. Conventional nonsurgical treatment based on mechanical debridement continues to be, as occurs in periodontics, the gold standard treatment [32, 39]. This is due to the fact that the bactericidal action of the laser is not capable of showing its efficacy without prior destructuring of the biofilm [26, 40]. Laser therapy therefore constitutes an aid to mechanical decontamination through thermal decontamination [40]. In a very similar way, it has also been shown that the use of the diode laser cannot replace the chemical disinfection obtained in endodontics with products such as sodium hypochlorite. In this way, it also constitutes an adjunctive treatment for the disinfection of the root canals [35].

3.2 Low-intensity photothermal therapy

3.2.1 Mechanism of action

Low-level light/laser therapy (LLLT) is the application of light (usually delivered via a low-power laser or light-emitting diode; LED) to promote tissue repair, reduce inflammation or induce analgesia [41]. The basis of low-intensity photothermal therapy is that its activity on tissues is not due to thermal effects but to the interaction of electromagnetic waves with cells [8]. This laser therapy uses the action of light and light alone to directly stimulate host cells in order to reduce inflammation, relieve pain and/or promote wound healing [41]. The therapy uses low-power lasers, also called soft lasers. These emit in the region of the infrared spectrum near red (632, 670 and 830 nm), with powers lower than 0,5 W or with lasers of higher emission power but used in defocused mode [9]. Its basic applications in health sciences are based on its tissue biostimulation effects and its anti-inflammatory analgesic action [42].

The mechanism of action of low-power laser therapy is based on cellular biostimulation. The photon-cell interaction mechanism consists of biomodulating tissue cells by supplying them with laser light, causing effects at a cellular level [43]. These effects occur due to the absorption of photons of a certain wavelength by the cellular photoreceptors, causing the transformation of the functional and metabolic activity of the cells [44]. In fact most of the effects of this biomodulation can be explained by light absorption within the mitochondria [41, 45].

The effect of photobiomodulation is based on its action on energy reserves in the adenosine triphosphate (ATP) in cells [45]. When the cell is damaged, these reserves decrease, and therefore, its metabolic activity is altered. The laser radiation acts directly on the photoreceptors of the respiratory chain, facilitating the conversion of adenosine diphosphate (ADP) to ATP [44]. Increased ATP stores facilitate the general activation of cellular metabolism. In turn, DNA is activated by ATP and protein synthesis begins, which results in the formation of structural proteins [41]. As laser radiation acts as an activator of protein synthesis and therefore of cell function, the processes of cell division and multiplication are accelerated [44]. This phenomenon could be responsible for the improvement in tissue healing when this therapy is used.

Laser energy is absorbed more easily where the concentration of fluids is greatest. Therefore, there will be a greater absorption in the inflamed and oedematous tissues, stimulating the numerous biological reactions related to the wound repair process [45]. Therefore, the biostimulatory effects of laser irradiation, such as higher cell proliferation and wound healing, may have interesting applications in current therapy approaches such as promotion of wound healing and reduction of inflammation as well as pain relief [41].

The effects of biostimulation by low-intensity laser therapy on cell metabolism are reflected at the clinical level. It has been documented that the activation and proliferation of human gingival fibroblasts, periodontal ligament cells, osteoblasts and mesenchymal stem cells, and the release of growth factors *in vitro*, were enhanced by low-level laser irradiation, according to several studies [16, 46, 47]. Reductions in inflammation have also been reported, and several *in vitro* studies indicated the reduction of proinflammatory molecules, such as prostaglandin E2, interleukins and tumour necrosis factor-alpha [48, 49]. Low-level laser therapy has been reported to promote osteogenesis, and several *in vitro* studies have shown that laser irradiation could promote bone nodule formation by inducing osteoblast proliferation and differentiation [50, 51]. This evidence has also been demonstrated in *in vivo* studies, and several histological studies indicated an increase in angiogenesis and the formation of connective tissue, also observing an increase in the formation of new bone in the site treated with laser, compared to the non-treated controls [52, 53].

3.2.2 Main indications

Dental applications for low-intensity photothermal therapy are not well documented; however, more studies are now being reported. In fact, we now have promising data for the application of this diode laser therapy in a number of dental specialities including endodontics, periodontics, orthodontics, and maxillofacial surgery, as described below [41].

In surgery, it can be used after especially complex extractions to reduce pain, oedema trismus, and inflammation. It can also be used to promote osteogenesis after tooth extraction because laser-irradiated extraction wound healing showed different characteristics from those of the normal healing process, suggesting the promotion of healing [54, 55]. In periodontics, the anti-inflammatory effect reduces the deterioration of periodontal tissues, reduces inflammation, and facilitates the hygienic phase, polished scaling and root planing or periodontal surgical treatments [56, 57]. In implant therapy, low-level laser therapy applied after conventional techniques shows promise for increased and faster osseointegration of implants following irradiation [16]. This therapy can also be useful in the treatment of peri-implant pathologies, since if it is used as an adjunct to conventional therapy [58], it could favour the reduction of inflammation and contribute to osteogenesis and tissue regeneration [41]. This treatment is shown in **Figure 2**.

Another important application of low-intensity photothermal therapy is in orthodontics. The essence of orthodontics is based on causing dental or orthopaedic movements by applying controlled forces. The use of laser has been studied to accelerate tooth movement by favouring bone remodelling due to its biostimulation effect, which allows orthodontic treatments to be performed in less time [59]. In addition, its anti-inflammatory and analgesic effect has proven to be effective, not only reducing treatment time but also reducing the pain and inflammation inherent to these types of treatment [60].

In oral pathology, this therapy is used for the stimulation of the physiological response of tissues. Its use in the treatment of various injuries has been described [46]. In the case of herpes simplex, soft lasers produce a similar effect to acyclovir, and it has been shown that if 2 J/cm^2 is applied in the prodromal phase, the blisters are likely to

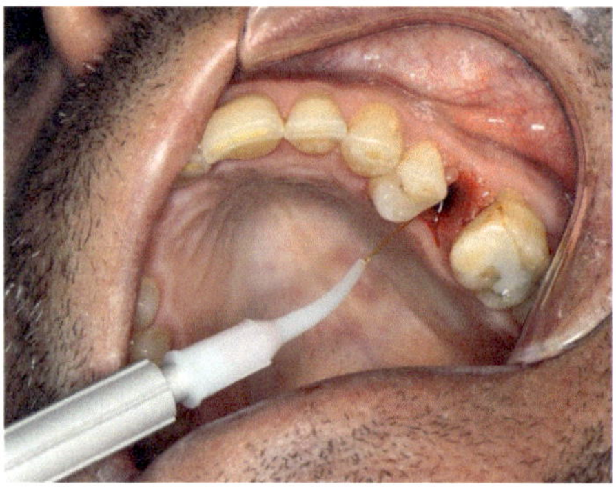

Figure 2.
Fox III 890 nm diode laser (a.R.C. Laser GmbH, Nürnberg, Germany) diffusor optical fibre tip being used in the treatment of peri-implant mucositis.

disappear in 2–3 days with little discomfort, instead of 8 to 14 days. Low-intensity laser therapy also appears to reduce the frequency of recurrence and the rate of relapse. The main advantages of herpes simplex laser treatment appear to be the absence of side effects and drug interactions, which are especially useful for older and immunocompromised patients [61]. It has also been documented in the management of herpes zoster, trigeminal neuralgia, and recurrent aphthous stomatitis [41, 62]. The diode laser acts as an analgesic relieving pain, and in some cases, such as canker sores, it also shortens the healing time [41]. Another important application in oral medicine is its use in oral mucositis, since these ulcerative-type oral lesions produced by radiotherapy or chemotherapy can compromise the quality of life and nutrition of patients. Diode lasers, in conjunction with low-intensity laser therapy, have been shown to reduce the severity of oral mucositis and can be used prophylactically before radiation. Once produced, the lesions provide an analgesic effect and accelerate healing (**Table 3**) [63].

3.2.3 Contraindications

The main contraindication of this therapy is its use in malignant or premalignant oral lesions. This is because cells with dysplasia have a higher metabolic activity and are much more sensitive to biostimulation from laser light. Irradiating these lesions with low-power lasers could worsen the degree of dysplasia and stimulate tumour growth [41]. Another limitation of this laser therapy is that, as occurred in high-intensity laser therapy, in some cases, it must be used as adjuvant therapy, and its use as replacement therapy is more

Oral Surgery	Periodontics	Implantology	Oral Pathology
• Third molar extraction • Paraesthesia alveolar nerve • Reduced pain, reduced swelling, improved trismus	• Coadjuvant treatment of periodontal disease • Reduced inflammation Improved healing	• Coadjuvant treatment of peri-implant pathologies • Osseointegration of dental implants • Reduced pain	• Herpes simplex • Herpes Zoster • Trigeminal neuralgia • Recurrent aphthous stomatitis • Oral mucositis • Temporomandibular disorders

Table 3.
Main indications in dentistry for low-intensity photothermal therapy.

limited, for example, in the treatment of periodontal disease or peri-implant pathologies [24]. However, even if it does not replace conventional therapies, it could have a coadjuvant effect that makes a difference in terms of pain management and inflammation.

4. Photodynamic or photochemical therapy

4.1 Mechanism of action

Photodynamic therapy is based on a non-thermal photochemical mechanism. This treatment aims to achieve the same bactericidal effects as high-intensity photothermal therapy but uses laser emission powers comparable to low-intensity photothermal therapy [40]. This is achieved thanks to the interaction of the laser light with the photosensitising pigment, and it is important to emphasise that temperature does not intervene in this interaction, only the absorption of the wavelength of the emitting laser by the photosensitiser [64].

The photodynamic process is therefore based on a photochemical reaction. A photochemical reaction is one in which light initiates a chemical process [65]. A pigment, called a photosensitiser, is used, which selectively reaches the cell or microorganism to be eliminated and is irradiated with a wavelength according to the selected pigment [40]. For this process to be carried out, the photosensitiser must be administered to the target and be irradiated with the specific wavelength; then, it reacts and produces reactive oxygen species (ROS) like hydroxyl radicals [64, 66]. These will cause oxidative stress that leads to damage or destruction of the cell membranes, causing irreversible biological damage. This damage will always be selective since only the selected microorganisms will be sensitive to the photosensitiser and therefore affected by this therapy [67].

In recent years, photodynamic therapy has proven to be an effective, noninvasive and highly specialised treatment alternative in bacterial elimination [68]. However, for the successful elimination of bacteria, some elements must be taken into account. As it is an oxygen-dependent process, its usefulness will be limited in areas poor in this element. In these cases, photothermal therapy can be a more effective option for bacterial elimination [65, 66].

Another key aspect is the choice of photosensitiser and the light source. In antimicrobial photodynamic therapy, it is essential that the photosensitiser has a high affinity for pathogenic microorganisms and also a low binding affinity with the cells of the host tissues [65, 69]. Most of the photosensitisers marketed in dentistry are made from Methylene Blue, Toluidine Blue, or some of their fractions. Another common photosensitiser used in recent years is indocyanine green solution [64]. Regarding the light source and laser parameters, these must be specific to activate the photosensitiser [66]. Various light sources have been used in the literature, such as helium-neon, diode and argon lasers activated by wavelengths between 630 and 810 nm [64]. However, other combinations of photosensitisers and wavelengths appear [67]. The important thing is to emphasise that there must always be an affinity between the photosensitiser and the wavelength with which it is irradiated in order for photodynamic therapy to be effective and safe [65].

4.2 Main indications

The general indications of photodynamic therapy are clear: to eliminate bacteria, fungi, viruses, or fungi resistant to other types of treatments. It is true that the photothermic effect produced by most high-power lasers can produce high decontamination of irradiated areas, but this can involve a high risk of damage to neighbouring structures in the contaminated area [64]. Photodynamic therapy is therefore postulated as a more conservative treatment.

Some of its main indications are in the speciality of periodontics and implantology. The central role of bacteria in the development of peri-implant pathologies and periodontal disease is well known [70]. Biofilms that colonise tooth surfaces and epithelial cells lining the periodontal pocket/gingival sulcus (subgingival dental plaques) are among the most complex biofilms that exist in nature [40]. Therapies that improve the results of conventional therapies based on mechanical debridement are constantly being sought [71]. Systemic use of antibiotics in conjunction with mechanical treatment is a commonly performed treatment modality in periodontology and is regarded as a reliable method in the treatment of periodontal diseases [72]. Photodynamic therapy has been suggested as an alternative to chemical antimicrobial agents and antibiotics to eliminate subgingival species [40]. Microbiological reduction was observed *in vivo* following photodynamic therapy in the treatment of peri-implantitis in animal model [73]. Also, it has been observed in randomised controlled trials that scaling and root planing, combined with photodisinfection, leads to a reduction of pocket depths, bleeding scores and clinical attachment gain in the nonsurgical treatment of periodontitis [74, 75]. However, other similar trials did not obtain statistically significant differences in the reduction of clinical parameters applying photodynamic diode laser therapy [12, 76]. Therefore, the potential effects of antimicrobial photodynamic therapy should be studied more extensively to establish the optimal conditions during clinical application [72] since recent systematic reviews and metanalysis such as the one published by Bashir et al. have reported promising results that encourage further research [77].

This therapy can also be used in restorative dentistry. Treatment of cavitated lesions involves the surgical removal of the infected tooth structure followed by tooth restoration [40]. The antibacterial capacity of the diode laser can be used once the cavity to be filled has been made, since the exposed dentin may contain, in addition to hydroxyapatite remains, odontoblastic extensions, collagen, and other common debris of the smear layer, bacteria typical of dentin infection [78]. Therefore, photodynamic therapy could be used as a minimally invasive technique to eliminate bacteria within carious lesions [40]. Several laboratory studies have demonstrated, using toluidine blue, the susceptibility of cariogenic bacteria to photodynamic therapy [78–80]. This technique could offer the following benefits: rapid noninvasive topical *in vivo* application of the drug to the carious lesion; rapid bacterial killing after a short exposure to light; unlikely development of resistance considering the widespread generic toxicity of reactive oxygen species; and confined killing by restricting the field of irradiation and the inherently short diffusion radius of reactive oxygen species [40].

Another speciality in which bacterial elimination is a central axis is endodontics. The ultimate goal of endodontic treatment is the elimination of infection from the root canal system [72]. For root canal treatments, irrigation solutions such as sodium hypochlorite are used, constituting a powerful chemical disinfection system that is difficult to overcome [81]. However, there are some situations, such as necrotic teeth with open apices, where hypochlorite irrigation can reach beyond the apex, penetrating the tissues adjacent to the apex and producing necrosis of said tissues. It is in these cases like this that photodynamic therapy can be used without risk of complications [40, 81]. It is true that activated photo disinfection is not higher than that produced

Periodontics	Implantology	Restorative	Endodontics
• Coadjuvant treatment of periodontal disease	• Coadjuvant treatment of peri-implant pathologies	• Disinfection of cavitated lesions	• Coadjuvant to root canal irrigation • Root canal irrigation with open apex

Table 4.
Main indications in dentistry for photodynamic therapy.

by hypochlorite, but the risk involved is much lower [72]. Photodynamic therapy has been employed in recent years to target microorganisms in root canals *in vitro* [82, 83] and *in vivo* [84, 85]. These studies suggested the potential of photodynamic therapy as an adjunctive technique to eliminate residual root canal bacteria after standard endodontic chemo-mechanical debridement [40]. Thus, in endodontics, the application of diode laser photodynamic therapy in specific cases can replace the use of sodium hypochlorite to improve the bactericidal effect during the biomechanical preparation of the root canal (**Table 4**) [81].

4.3 Contraindications

For a successful bacterial photoelimination, some factors must be considered, e.g., the selection of appropriate photosensitiser, light source and parameters [64]. The microorganisms to be eliminated must be known, as well as the characteristics of the photosensitiser and the wavelength to which it responds. If the pigment does not bind to the microorganisms, it is used in excess or insufficient quantity, or it is not irradiated with the specified wavelength, the therapy will not achieve good results [81].

Photosensitisers are not universal, and although they are capable of acting on a wide variety of microorganisms, some may not be affected. Another limitation is that bacteria associate to form dynamic structures called biofilms [72]. This structure, where a great variety of bacteria coexist, prevents the photosensitiser from penetrating deeply, with which the bactericidal effect may not be complete. It has been suggested, in studies of model systems, that water channels can carry solutes into or out of the depths of a biofilm, but they do not guarantee access to the interior of the cell clusters [40, 77]. For this reason, we need to deconstruct the biofilm before using this laser therapy, as happened in photothemic therapies [77].

5. Future research lines with diode laser

Diode laser technology and its different applications in dentistry date back several decades; however, it has been in the last 10 years that it has gained a greater prominence thanks to the great technical development achieved and the materialisation of affordable equipment for the dentist. All this advancement has allowed it to be used today in many procedures to improve the performance of conventional therapies and yet this is not enough. The use of different diode laser therapies should be consolidated with more research. In recent years, progress has been made in this regard as it has gained more and more prominence as adjuvant therapy; however, although there are several important *in vitro* [29, 86, 87] and clinical studies [66, 74, 75, 88], more research is still needed to address laser therapy from a different perspective.

More research is needed to study the different diode laser therapies from a histological, immunological and microbiological point of view [77]. The contemporary notion of how oral biofilms are causing oral diseases, such as tooth decay, periodontitis, or peri-implantitis, is well summarised by the "ecological plaque hypothesis". According to this hypothesis, it is the interrelation between the bacteria and the host's response that defines health or disease [89]. Current treatment techniques involve either periodic mechanical disruption of oral microbial biofilms or maintaining therapeutic concentrations of antimicrobials in the oral cavity, both of which are fraught with limitations [40].

We know that the true potential of the diode laser lies in its bactericidal capacity, either through temperature or photosensitisation, and in its ability to stimulate the host's immune response against that aggression. Therefore, studies are needed to provide the scientific community with evidence of this potential. Microbiological studies compare the bacterial reduction between conventional therapies and the adjuvant use of diode laser, immunological studies correlate this bacterial decrease with the activation of the host's immune system, and histological studies show how areas irradiated with diode laser heal better and with less pain and inflammation than those that have not been treated with laser. In summary, more high-quality, randomised controlled trials are necessitated before recommendations for use can be made [40, 72, 77]; only when we consolidate this knowledge will we be able to understand the clinical effects of diode laser therapies.

6. Conclusions

Diode laser therapies have shown promising results in dentistry. For our discipline, its potential lies in its bactericidal and biostimulation capacity. However, due to the complex field of application that is the oral cavity, more high-quality, randomised controlled trials with good methodology are necessary to show the true efficacy of these therapies, studies that evaluate the diode laser not only from a clinical perspective but also from a microbiological and immunological point of view. With solid scientific evidence, even today under construction, in the future, clinical protocols could be achieved. Therefore, it is now the time to investigate and demonstrate clear evidence of clinical efficacy and applicability to show the true potential of diode laser therapies in destintry.

Acknowledgements

The authors would like to thank the Faculty of Health Sciences from Universidad Europea de Valencia for their help with this book chapter.

Conflict of interest

The authors declare that they have no conflicts of interest.

Author details

Santiago Arias-Herrera*, Rebeca Sánchez-Martos and Lourdes Alfaro-Ochoa
Faculty of Health Sciences, Department of Dentistry, Universidad Europea de Valencia, Valencia, Spain

*Address all correspondence to: santiagoemilio.arias@universidadeuropea.es

References

[1] Wheeland RG. Clinical use of laser in dermatology. Laser in Surgery and Medicine. 1995;**16**:2-23

[2] España-Tost AJ, Arnabat-Domínguez J, Berini-Aytés L, Gay-Escoda C. Aplicaciones del láser en Odontología. RCOE. 2004;**9**:497-511

[3] Sargaiyan V, Yadan R, Parihar S, Sapat M, SLA B. Lasers in dentistry. International Journal of Preventive and Clinical Dental Research. 2017;**4**:304-307

[4] Maiman TH. Stimulated optical radiation in ruby. Nature. 1960;**187**:493

[5] Stern RH, Sognnaes RF. Laser beam effect on dental hard tissue. Journal of Dental Research. 1964;**43**:873

[6] Goldman L, Gray JA, Goldman J, Goldman B, Meyer R. Effect of laser beam impacts on teeth. Journal of the American Dental Association. 1965;**70**:601

[7] Kinersly T, Jarabak JP, Phatak NM, DeMent J. Laser effects on tissue and materials related to dentistry. Journal of the American Dental Association. 1965;**70**:593

[8] Green J, Weiss ASA. Lasers and radiofrequency devices in dentistry. Dental Clinics of North America. 2011;**55**:585-597

[9] Convissar RA. The biologic rationale for the use of lasers in dentistry. Dental Clinics of North America. 2004;**48**:771-794

[10] Dederich D, Busshick R. Lasers in dentistry: Separating science from hype. Journal of the American Dental Association (1939). 2004;**135**:204-212

[11] Strauss R. Lasers in oral and maxillofacial surgery. Dental Clinics of North America. 2004;**4**:851-871

[12] Andersen R, Loebel N, Hammond D, Wilson M. Treatment of periodontal disease by photo-disinfection compared to scaling and root planing. The Journal of Clinical Dentistry. 2007;**18**:34-38

[13] Wilson M, Dobson J, Sarkar S. Sensitization of periodonto- pathogenic bacteria to killing by light from a low-power laser. Oral Microbiology and Immunology. 1993;**8**:182-187

[14] Garg A. Lasers in dental implantology: Innovation improves patient care. Dental Implantology Update. 2007;**18**:57-61

[15] Garg H, Garg V. Peri implantitis and lasers: A review. International Journal of Biological & Medical Research. 2012;**3**:2302-2305

[16] Aoki A, Mizutani K, Schwarz F, Sculean A, Yukna RA, Takasaki AA, et al. Periodontal and periimplant wound healing following laser therapy. Periodontology 2000. 2000;**2015**(68):217-269

[17] Kato J, Moriya K, Jayawardena JA, Wijeye-weera RL, Awazu K. Prevention of dental caries in partially erupted permanent teeth with a CO_2 laser. Journal of Clinical Laser Medicine & Surgery. 2003;**21**:369-374

[18] Deppe H, Horch H. Laser applications in oral surgery and implant dentistry. Lasers in Medical Science. 2007;**22**:217-221

[19] Perveen A, Molardi C, Fornaini C. Applications of laser welding in

dentistry: A state of the art review. Micromachines (Basel). 2018;**9**(5):209

[20] Aoki A, Mizutani K, Takasaki AA, Sasaki KM, Nagai S, Schwarz F, et al. Current status of clinical laser applications in periodontal therapy. General Dentistry. 2008;**56**:674-687

[21] Mizutani K, Aoki A, Coluzzi D, Yukna R, Wang CY. Lasers in minimally invasive periodontal and peri-implant therapy. Periodontology 2000. 2000;**2016**(71):185-212

[22] Weiner GP. Laser dentistry practice management. Dental Clinics of North America. 2004;**48**:1105-1126

[23] Pang P, Andreana S, Aoki S, Coluzzi D, Obeidi A, Olivi G, et al. Laser energy in oral soft tissue applications: Position paper. Journal of Laser Dentistry. 2010;**18**:123-131

[24] Romanos G, Nentwig GH. Diode laser (980 nm) in oral and maxillofacial surgical procedures: Clinical observations based on clinical applications. Journal of Clinical Laser Medicine & Surgery. 1999;**17**:193-197

[25] Cobb CM. Lasers in periodontics: A review of the literature. Journal of Periodontology. 2006;**77**:545-564

[26] Ishikawa I, Aoki A, Takasaki A, Mizutani K, Izumi Y. Application of lasers in periodontics: True innovation or myth? Periodontology 2000. 2000;**2009**(50):90-126

[27] Cobb C, Low S, Coluzzi D. Lasers and the treatment of chronic periodontitis. Dental Clinics of North America. 2010;**54**:35-53

[28] Schwarz F, Sculean A, Berakdar M, Szathmari L, Georg T, Becker J. *In vivo* and *in vitro* effects of an Er: YAG laser, a GaAlAs diode laser, and scaling and root planing on periodontally diseased root surfaces: A comparative histologic study. Lasers in Surgery and Medicine. 2003;**32**:359-366

[29] Assaf M, Yilmaz S, Kuru B, Ipci SD, Noyun U, Kadir T. Effect of the diode laser on bacteremia associated with dental ultrasonic scaling: A clinical and microbiological study. Photomedicine and Laser Surgery. 2007;**25**:250-256

[30] Zitzmann N, Berglundh T. Definition and prevalence of peri- implant diseases. Journal of Clinical Periodontology. 2008;**35**:286-291

[31] Salvi GE, Sculean A, Lang NP, Ramseier CA. Reversibility of experimental peri-implant mucositis compared with experimental gingivitis in humans. Clinical Oral Implants Research. 2011;**23**:182-190

[32] Berglundh T, Armitage G, Araujo MG, Avila G, Blanco J, Camargo PM, et al. Peri - implant diseases and conditions: Consensus report of workgroup 4 of the 2017 world workshop on the classification of periodontal and peri - implant diseases and conditions. Journal of Clinical Periodontology. 2018;**45**:286-291

[33] Romanos GE, Everts H, Nentwig GH. Effects of diode and Nd: YAG laser irradiation on titanium discs: A scanning electron microscope examination. Journal of Periodontology. 2000;**71**:810-815

[34] Matsumoto K. Lasers in endodontics. Dental Clinics of North America. 2000;**4**:889-905

[35] Saydjari Y, Kuypers T, Gutknecht N. Laser application in dentistry: Irradiation effects of Nd:YAG 1064 nm and diode 810 nm and 980 nm in infected root

canals: A literature overview. Biomedical Research. 2016;**2016**:8421656

[36] Beer F, Buchmair A, Wernisch J, Georgopoulos A, Moritz A. Comparison of two diode lasers on bactericidity in root canals an *in vitro* study. Lasers in Medical Science. 2012;**27**:361-364

[37] Walling J, Kirchhoff T, Berthold M, Wenzler JS, Braun A. Impact of thermal photodynamic disinfection on root dentin temperature *in vitro*. Photodiagnosis and Photodynamic Therapy. 2021;**35**:102476

[38] Moritz A, Gutknecht N, Goharkhay K, Schoop U, Wernisch J, Sperr W. *In vitro* irradiation of infected root canals with a diode laser: Results of microbiologic, infrared spectrometric, and stain penetration examinations. Quintessence International. 1997;**28**:205-209

[39] Heitz-mayfield LJA, Salvi GE. Peri-implant mucositis. Journal of Periodontology. 2018;**20**:S237-S245

[40] Soukos NS, Goodson JM. Photodynamic therapy in the control of oral biofilms. Periodontology 2000. 2011;**55**(1):143-166

[41] Carrolla JD, Milwardb MR, Cooperb PR, Hadisc M, Palin W. Developments in low level light therapy (LLLT) for dentistry. Dental Materials. 2014;**30**:465-475

[42] Smith K. The photobiological basis of low level laser therapy. Laser Therapy. 1991;**3**:19-24

[43] Chung H, Dai T, Sharma SK, Huang YY, Carroll JD, Hamblin MR. The nuts and bolts of low-level laser (light) therapy. Annals of Biomedical Engineering. 2012;**40**:516-533

[44] Sommer A. Revisiting the photon/cell interaction mechanism in low-level light therapy. Photobiomodulation, Photomedicine, and Laser Surgery. 2019;**37**:336-341

[45] Karu TI. Mitochondrial mechanisms of photobiomodulation in context of new data about multiple roles of ATP. Photomedicine and Laser Surgery. 2010;**28**:159-160

[46] Almeida-Lopes L, Rigau J, Zangaro RA, Guidugli-Neto J, Jaeger MM. Comparison of the low level laser therapy effects on cultured human gingival fibroblasts proliferation using different irradiance and same fluence. Lasers in Surgery and Medicine. 2001;**29**:179-184

[47] Khadra M, Lyngstadaas SP, Haanaes HR, Mustafa K. Effect of laser therapy on attachment, proliferation and differentiation of human osteoblast like cells cultured on titanium implant material. Biomaterials. 2005;**26**:3503-3509

[48] Gavish L, Perez LS, Reissman P, Gertz SD. Irradiation with 780 nm diode laser attenuates inflammatory cytokines but upregulates nitric oxide in lipopolysaccharide stimulated macrophages: Implications for the prevention of aneurysm progression. Lasers in Surgery and Medicine. 2008;**40**:371-378

[49] Sakurai Y, Yamaguchi M, Abiko Y. Inhibitory effect of low- level laser irradiation on LPS-stimulated prostaglandin E2 production and cyclooxygenase-2 in human gingival fibroblasts. European Journal of Oral Sciences. 2000;**108**:29-34

[50] Ozawa Y, Shimizu N, Kariya G, Abiko Y. Low-energy laser irradiation stimulates bone nodule formation at early stages of cell culture in rat calvarial cells. Bone. 1998;**22**:347-354

[51] Stein A, Benayahu D, Maltz L, Oron U. Low-level laser irradiation promotes proliferation and differentiation of human osteoblasts *in vitro*. Photomedicine and Laser Surgery. 2005;**23**:161-166

[52] Merli LA, Santos MT, Genovese WJ, Faloppa F. Effect of low-intensity laser irradiation on the process of bone repair. Photomedicine and Laser Surgery. 2005;**23**:212-215

[53] Pinheiro AL, Limeira Junior Fde A, Gerbi ME, Ramalho LM, Marzola C, Ponzi EA, et al. Effect of 830-nm laser light on the repair of bone defects grafted with inorganic bovine bone and decalcified cortical osseus membrane. Journal of Clinical Laser Medicine & Surgery. 2003;**21**:301-306

[54] Pejcic A, Kojovic D, Kesic L, Obradovic R. The effects of low level laser irradiation on gingival inflammation. Photomedicine and Laser Surgery. 2010;**28**:69-74

[55] Markovic AB, Todorovic L. Postoperative analgesia after lower third molar surgery: Contribution of the use of long-acting local anesthetics, low-power laser and diclofenac. Oral Surgery, Oral Medicine, Oral Pathology, Oral Radiology, and Endodontics. 2006;**102**(102):e4-e8

[56] Ozawa Y, Shimizu N, Abiko. Low-energy diode laser irradiation reduced plasminogen activator activity in human periodontal ligament cells. Lasers in Surgery and Medicine. 1997;**21**:456-463

[57] Makhlouf M, Dahaba MM, Tunér J, Eissa SA, Harhash TA. Effect of adjunctive low level laser therapy (LLLT) on nonsurgical treatment of chronic periodontitis. Photomedicine and Laser Surgery. 2012;**30**:160-166

[58] Sánchez-Martos R, Samman A, Bouazza-Juanes K, Díaz-Fernández J-M, Arias-Herrera S. Clinical effect of diode laser on peri-implant tissues during non-surgical peri-implant mucositis therapy: Randomized controlled clinical study. Journal of Clinical and Experimental Dentistry. 2020;**12**:e13-e21

[59] Genc G, Kocadereli I, Tasar F, Kilinc K, El S, Sarkarati B. Effect of low-level laser therapy (LLLT) on orthodontic tooth movement. Lasers in Medical Science. 2013;**28**:41-47

[60] Yang JZ, K. Clinical research: Low-level laser therapy in accelerating orthodontic tooth movement. BMC Oral Health. 2021;**21**:324

[61] Eduardo CP, Aranha AC, Simoes A, Bello-Silva MS, Ramalho KM, Esteves-Oliveira M, et al. Laser treatment of recurrent herpes labialis: A literature review. Lasers in Medical Science. 2012;**29**:1517-1529

[62] De Souza TO, Martins MA, Bussadori SK, Fernandes KP, Tanji EY, Mesquita-Ferrari RA, et al. Clinical evaluation of LLLT for recurring aphtous stomatitis. Photomedicine and Laser Surgery. 2010;**28**:S85-S88

[63] Simões A, Eduardo FP, Luiz AC, Campos L, Cristófaro M, Marques MM, et al. Laser phototherapy as topical prophylaxis against head and neck cancer radiotherapy induced oral mucositis: Comparison between low and high/low power lasers. Lasers in Surgery and Medicine. 2009;**41**:264-270

[64] Fekrazada R, Khoeib F, Hakimiha N, Bahador A. Photoelimination of *Streptococcus mutans* with two methods of photodynamic and photothermal therapy. Photodiagnosis and Photodynamic Therapy. 2013;**10**:626-631

[65] Salvi GE, Stähli A, Schmidt JC, Ramseier CA, Sculean A, Walter C. Adjunctive laser or antimicrobial photodynamic therapy to non-surgical mechanical instrumentation in patients with untreated periodontitis: A systematic review and meta-analysis. Journal of Clinical Periodontology. 2020;**47**:176-198

[66] Hill G, Dehn C, Hinze AV, Frentzen M, Meister J. Indocyanine green-based adjunctive antimicrobial photodynamic therapy for treating chronic periodontitis: A randomized clinical trial. Photodiagnosis and Photodynamic Therapy. 2019;**26**:29-35

[67] Fekrazad R, Karamifar K, Bahador A. Comparison of antibacterial effect of photodynamic therapy using indocyanine green (Emundo) with 2% metronidazole and 2% chlorhexidine gel on *Porphyromonas gingivalis* (an *in-vitro* study). Photodiagnosis and Photodynamic Therapy. 2016;**15**:28-33

[68] Takeuchi Y, Aoki A, Hiratsuka K, Chui C, Ichinose A, Aung N, et al. Application of different wavelengths of LED lights in antimicrobial photodynamic therapy for the treatment of periodontal disease. Antibiotics (Basel). 2023;**28**(12):1676

[69] Katsikanis F, Strakas D, Vouros I. The application of antimicrobial photodynamic therapy (aPDT, 670 nm) and diode laser (940 nm) as adjunctive approach in the conventional cause-related treatment of chronic periodontal disease: A randomized controlled split-mouth clinical trial. Clinical Oral Investigations. 2020;**24**(5):1821-1827

[70] Caton J, Armitage G, Berglundh T, Chapple IL, Jepsen S, Kornman K, et al. A new classification scheme for periodontal and periimplant diseases and conditions – Introduction and key changes from the 1999 classification. Journal of Clinical Periodontology. 2018;**45**:S1-S8

[71] Sánchez-Martos R, Samman A, Priami M, Arias-Herrera S. The diode laser as coadyuvant therapy in the non-surgical conventional treatment of peri-implant mucositis: A systematic review and meta-analysis. Journal of Clinical and Experimental Dentistry. 2020;**12**(12):e1171-e1182

[72] Gursoy H, Ozcakir-Tomruk C, Tanalp J, Yilmaz S. Photodynamic therapy in dentistry: A literature review. Clinical Oral Investigations. 2012;**17**:1113-1125

[73] Komerik N, Nakanishi H, Robert MAJ, Henderson B, Wilson M. *In vivo* killing of *Porphyromonas gingivalis* by toluidine blue photosensitization in an animal model. Antimicrobial Agents and Chemotherapy. 2013;**47**:932-940

[74] Chondros P, Nikolidakis D, Christodoulides N, Rossler R, Gutknecht N, Sculean A. Photodynamic therapy as adjunct to non-surgical periodontal treatment in patients on periodontal maintenance: A randomized controlled clinical trial. Lasers in Medical Science. 2009;**24**:681-688

[75] Christodoulides N, Nikolidakis D, Chondros P, Becker J, Schwarz F, Rössler R, et al. Photodynamic therapy as an adjunct to non-surgical periodontal treatment: A randomized controlled clinical trial. Journal of Periodontology. 2008;**79**:1638-1644

[76] Polansky R, Haas M, Heschl A, Wimmer G. Clinical effectiveness of photodynamic therapy in the treatment of periodontitis. Journal of Clinical Periodontology. 2009;**36**:575-580

[77] Bashir NZ, Singh HA, Virdee S. Indocyanine green–mediated

antimicrobial photodynamic therapy as an adjunct to periodontal therapy: A systematic review and meta-analysis. Clinical Oral Investigations. 2021;**25**:5699-5710

[78] Giusti JS, Santos-Pinto L, Pizzolito AC, Helmerson K, Carvalho-Filho E, Kurachi C, et al. Antimicrobial photodynamic action on dentin using a light-emitting diode light source. Photomedicine and Laser Surgery. 2008;**26**:281-287

[79] Zanin IC, Goncalves RB, Junior AB, Hope CK, Pratten J. Susceptibility of *Streptococcus mutans* biofilms to photodynamic therapy: An *in vitro* study. The Journal of Antimicrobial Chemotherapy. 2005;**56**:324-330

[80] Zanin IC, Lobo MM, Rodrigues LK, Pimenta LA, Hofling JF, Goncalves RB. Photosensitization of *in vitro* biofilms by toluidine blue O combined with a light-emitting diode. European Journal of Oral Sciences. 2006;**114**:64-69

[81] Abdelkarim-Elafifi H, Parada-Avendaño I, Arnabat-Dominguez J. Photodynamic therapy in endodontics: A helpful tool to combat antibiotic resistance? A literature review. Antibiotics. 2021;**10**:1106-1114

[82] Fimple JL, Fontana CR, Foschi F, Ruggiero K, Song TC, et al. Photodynamic treatment of endodontic polymicrobial infection *in vitro*. Journal of Endodontia. 2008;**34**:728-734

[83] Fonseca MB, Junior PO, Pallota RC, Filho HF, Denardin OV, Rapoport A, et al. Photodynamic therapy for root canals infected with *Enterococcus faecalis*. Photomedicine and Laser Surgery. 2008;**26**:209-213

[84] Pinheiro SL, Schenka AA, Neto AA, de Souza CP, Rodriguez HM, Ribeiro MC. Photodynamic therapy in endodontic treatment of deciduous teeth. Lasers in Medical Science. 2009;**24**:521-526

[85] Garcez AS, Nunez SC, Hamblin MR, Ribeiro MS. Antimicrobial effects of photodynamic therapy on patients with necrotic pulps and periapical lesion. Journal of Endodontia. 2008;**34**:138-142

[86] Seal GJ, Spratt D, Bhatti M, Gulabivala K. An *in vitro* comparison of the bactericidal efficacy of lethal photosensitization or sodium hyphochlorite irrigation on *Streptococcus intermedius* biofilms in root canals. International Endodontic Journal. 2002;**35**:268-274

[87] Dörtbudak O, Haas R, Bernhart T, Mailath-Pokorny G. Lethal photosensitization for decontamination of implant surfaces in the treatment of peri-implantitis. Clinical Oral Implants Research. 2001;**12**:104-108

[88] Gandhi KK, Pavaskar R, Cappetta EG, Drew HJ. Effectiveness of adjunctive use of low-level laser therapy and photodynamic therapy after scaling and root planing in patients with chronic periodontitis. International Journal of Periodontics & Restorative Dentistry. 2020;**39**:837-843

[89] Belibasakis GN. Microbiological and immuno-pathological aspects of peri-implant diseases. Archives of Oral Biology. 2014;**59**:66-72

Chapter 7

Minimally Invasive, Non-Surgical Periodontal Treatment: Scaling and Root Planing

Luis V. Maita Véliz, Luis M. Maita Castañeda and María M. Castañeda Mosto

Abstract

Periodontal diseases are prevalent worldwide, affecting individuals of all ages, including children. Despite advances in scientific knowledge, these diseases still lead to significant tooth loss. Furthermore, research has shown a close link between periodontal diseases and systemic conditions such as respiratory and cardiological issues, hormonal imbalances, pregnancy complications, and more. Preventive measures and campaigns targeting periodontal health could yield significant results if implemented widely across different regions. It is imperative to extend such initiatives to children and adolescents, considering the high prevalence of periodontal diseases globally. Introducing early education on the importance of periodontal health could further reinforce preventive efforts and contribute to better quality of life in the future. In the current context, professionals can apply minimally invasive non-surgical periodontal therapy procedures to effectively manage these diseases in their early and moderate stages, leveraging the excellent repair capacity of periodontal tissues. Emphasizing proper hygiene practices is also essential.

Keywords: periodontal disease, biofilm, dental calculus, dental scaling, root planing

1. Introduction

Periodontal diseases have existed since the early stages of human civilization. Historical evidence suggests that periodontal disease existed as far back as 3000 years BC, among civilizations such as the Sumerians, who were known to practice dental hygiene using gold toothpicks. Similar evidence of periodontal diseases has been found in ancient Egypt, Greece, Peru [1–3], and other regions (**Figures 1** and **2**).

In modern times, periodontal diseases are recognized as a universal health issue affecting populations worldwide. Scientific evidence supports the effectiveness of scaling and root planing procedures in treating periodontal disease.

The treatment of periodontal inflammatory lesions is multifaceted, with the primary goals being their control and elimination. Therapeutic approaches consider factors such as the severity of the disease, individual patient needs, and relevant risk factors. By addressing these factors systematically, healthcare providers can achieve the best possible treatment outcomes [4, 5].

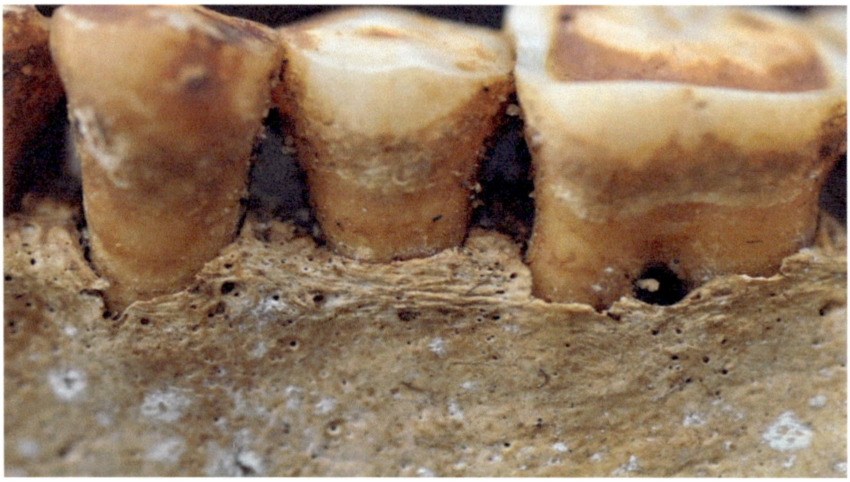

Figure 1.
Courtesy of Anton Samplonius. Jaw of an ancient Peruvian. Bone loss up to the middle third is observed in tooth 3.4. In tooth 3.5, the bone loss covers the cervical third of the root. In tooth 3.6, bone loss is observed in the mesial and distal roots and reaches the cervical third. The furcation presents a "tunnel"-type lesion that advances to the lingual surface.

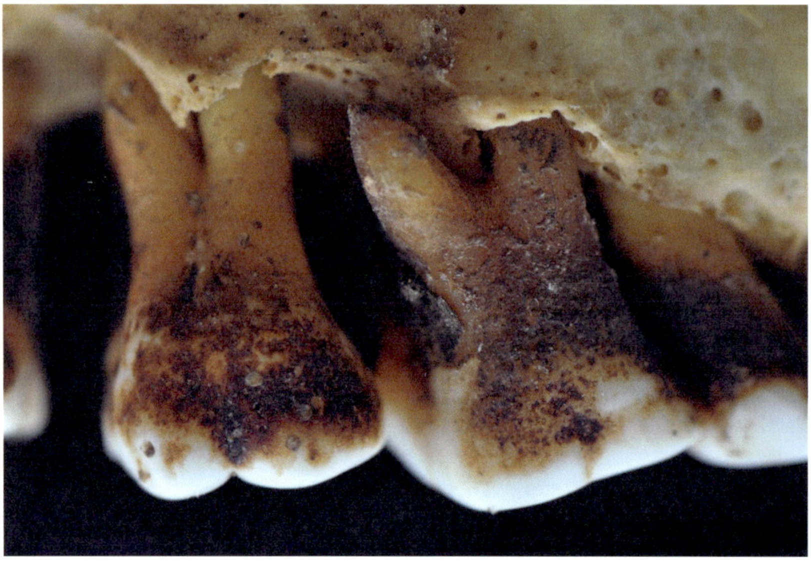

Figure 2.
Courtesy of Anton Samplonius. Upper jaw of an ancient Peruvian. Tooth 2.6 shows extensive bone loss from mesial to distal, reaching the apical third. In piece 2.7, we note that the bone loss is very extensive and has reached the mesial and distal roots. In the mesial root, it affects the apical third. The furcation area of this piece shows bone resorption. The presence of calculus in the molars is also observed. In tooth 2.6 the stone reaches the apex of the mesial root.

Non-surgical periodontal treatment is recommended for conditions such as gingivitis, gingival enlargements, and initial or moderate periodontitis. In such cases, the primary objective is to suppress local irritating factors [6–8].

However, it is important to note that non-surgical periodontal treatment may have limitations, particularly in interproximal areas or cases of bifurcation and trifurcation compromises, deep pockets, teeth in poor position, and intrabony defects [6].

2. Etiology of periodontal disease

The transition from health to disease occurs when specific bacteria within the bacterial biofilm proliferate and produce virulence factors that exceed the person's limit of defensive resistance. This can result from a decrease in the host's defenses, an exaggerated inflammatory response to bacterial attack, or the characteristics of the offending bacterial species, leading to the development of gingivitis or periodontitis and subsequent periodontal tissue destruction within a multifactorial pathogenic mechanism [9, 10].

The subgingival biofilm exhibits continuous presence and poses challenges for eradication, compounded by its constant exposure to gingival crevicular fluid (GCF). During inflammation, various cells and inflammatory biomarkers (enzymes, tissue degradation products, cytokines, etc.) are released into the GCF, necessitating analysis of its protein composition for predicting, diagnosing, and monitoring periodontal tissue health [11, 12].

Gram-negative bacteria within the biofilm continually release pro-inflammatory molecules such as bacterial lipopolysaccharides (LPS), which are endotoxins, and butyric acid. These bioactive substances interact with gingival tissue, initiating and amplifying the inflammatory response. Upon contacting the gingival epithelium, they can penetrate the connective tissue and enter the systemic circulation, emphasizing the importance of physically disrupting the biofilm to stop its growth.

Based on these principles, scaling and root planing are considered the "gold standard" of periodontal therapy for patients diagnosed with gingivitis, as well as those with initial and moderate periodontitis [13, 14]. In other words, non-surgical mechanical treatment is the cornerstone of periodontal therapy and the primary method recommended for controlling periodontal infections [15, 16].

3. Biofilm control

Non-surgical periodontal treatment must begin by empowering the patient to take control of the biofilm. This involves providing the patient with all the necessary information about the significance of biofilm control and educating them on effective periodontal hygiene techniques, including the selection of an appropriate toothbrush for biofilm removal.

When inflammation is confined to the gingival tissues, the treatment procedure primarily involves the removal of the biofilm using the proper periodontal hygiene techniques.

Figures 3–5 clearly illustrate the explanation given by the professional and demonstrate the application of scientific knowledge on biofilm control by the patient. These figures highlight the relatively simple procedures patients can undertake to achieve the benefits of periodontal health.

The fundamental procedure in combating periodontal infections remains the elimination of both supragingival and subgingival bacterial deposits.

The removal of supragingival plaque is crucial, as its presence can lead to the initial formation of subgingival plaque [17]. Supragingival plaque is composed primarily of gram-positive cocci and streptococci, which are aerobic bacteria and considered nonspecific opportunistic pathogens that induce gingivitis [18, 19].

Studies have shown that meticulous control of supragingival plaque can have a significant impact on both the quantity and quality of the subgingival microbiota, as

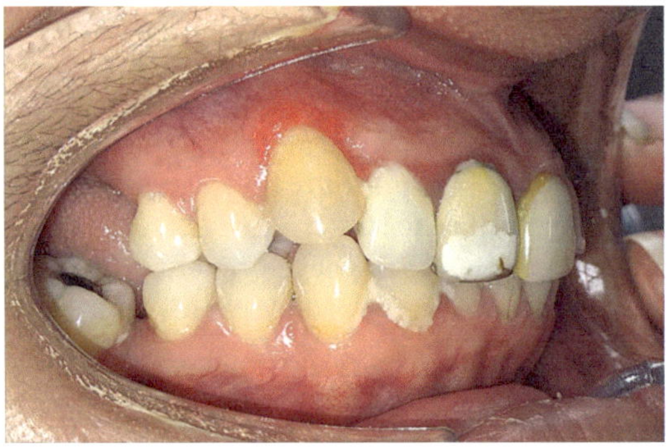

Figure 3.
In tooth 1.3 an inflammatory process is observed in the marginal gingiva and in a part of the attached gingiva.

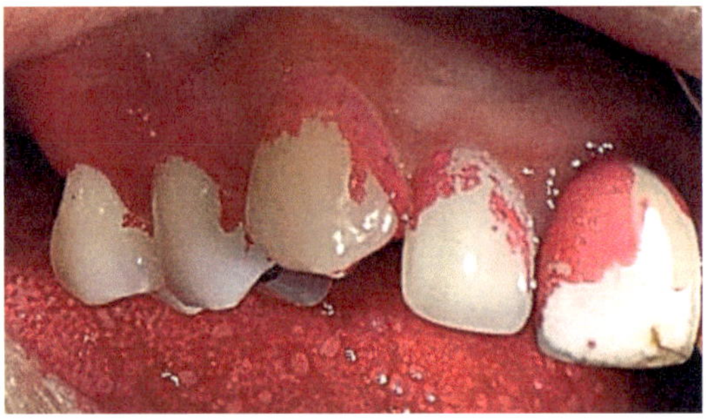

Figure 4.
The biofilm has taken on a greater extent in the cervical third of tooth 1.3 and in the neighboring teeth.

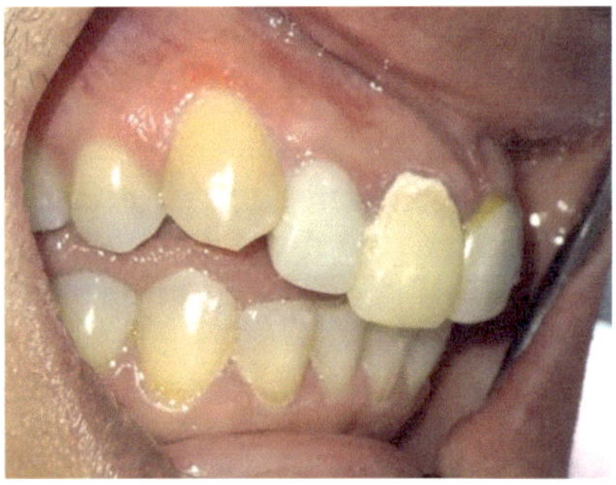

Figure 5.
The gingival inflammation of tooth 1.3 has been significantly reduced in just 21 days using the Modified Bass Technique.

well as the clinical symptoms associated with periodontitis in adults. This is because the quantity, composition, and recolonization rate of subgingival plaque are, to some extent, dependent on the accumulation of supragingival plaque [20–22].

4. Scaling and root planning

Scaling is defined as the procedure that removes the biofilm and dental calculus from the periodontal pocket, without modifying the root surface (**Figures 6** and 7).

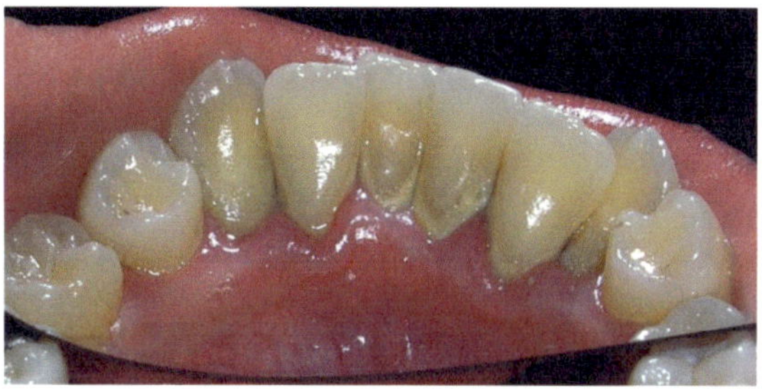

Figure 6.
Supragingival and subgingival calculus accumulation in the anterior region of the lingual surfaces of the incisors and canines.

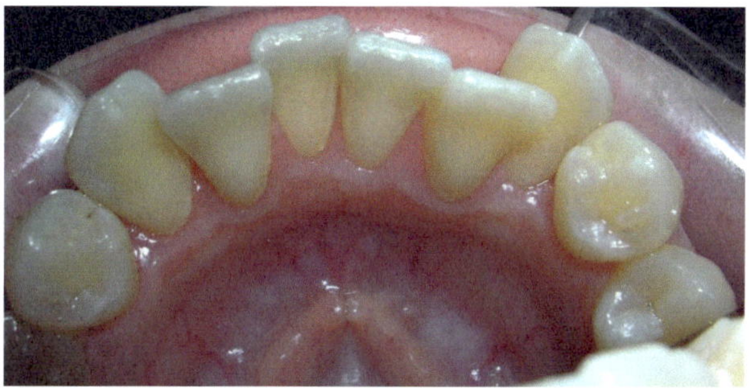

Figure 7.
Recovery of the gingival tissues can be seen after the removal of dental calculus from the anterior region of the lingual surfaces of the incisors and canines.

Scaling is carried out using mainly ultrasonic and manual methods.

The objective of this supragingival and subgingival mechanical debridement is to reduce the bacterial load, alter the microbial composition, and establish a flora that benefits the person's health. These microbiological changes help reduce inflammation and promote the stability of the periodontal attachment level [23].

In this chapter, we present our experience of scaling and root planing in clinical practice to show that these two procedures are the most important and fundamental in the treatment of bacterial periodontal diseases. While choosing a form of periodontal treatment is crucial, it does not singularly determine treatment success [24].

The success of periodontal treatments depends on several factors, including meticulous actions on the root surface of the teeth, patient compliance with periodontal maintenance, and consistent periodontal hygiene practices [25, 26]. A primary goal is the complete removal of subgingival calculus and biofilm.

Research indicates a significant reduction in subgingival bacterial load and specific periodontal pathogens following scaling and root planing in periodontitis [27]. Achieving thorough debridement of subgingival areas requires proper periodontal instruments, excellent technique, and training to prevent bacterial repopulation and reinfection due to residual calculus and biofilm [28].

While scaling and root planing are remarkably effective for reducing inflammation and reaching periodontal probing depths, subgingival calculus may remain inadvertently. Therefore, professionals recognize the importance of refining scaling and root planning techniques. These procedures are often clinically complex and resemble flapless periodontal surgery, requiring tactile perception similar to that of an open flap procedure.

Based on our clinical experience, we recommend the use of Hirshfield files and diamond tips (see **Figures 8** and **9**), which have proven highly effective in reaching inaccessible areas.

Preventing recurrence during periodontal requires meticulous scaling and root planing procedures and ongoing maintenance phases. Hirshfield files, particularly 3/7 (buccal and lingual) and 5/7 (mesial and distal), are very useful for non-surgical periodontal treatment. Before starting periodontal work, it is necessary to verify that the instruments have the necessary sharpness to be effective.

During treatment, the active part of the instrument must adapt to the root surface environment to remove subgingival calculus and biofilm without causing unnecessary trauma to soft tissues. Movements typically include vertical, oblique and, occasionally, horizontal motions. Every five movements, it is crucial to check for the presence of subgingival calculus and ensure its total removal [29].

When root surfaces become smoother, using a periodontal probe followed by tactile verification with a periodontal file helps identify any remaining roughness requiring further treatment. Incomplete removal of subgingival calculus can result in bacterial reservoirs, as spaces and channels within the stones allow bacterial proliferation and toxin accumulation, along with other microorganisms [30, 31].

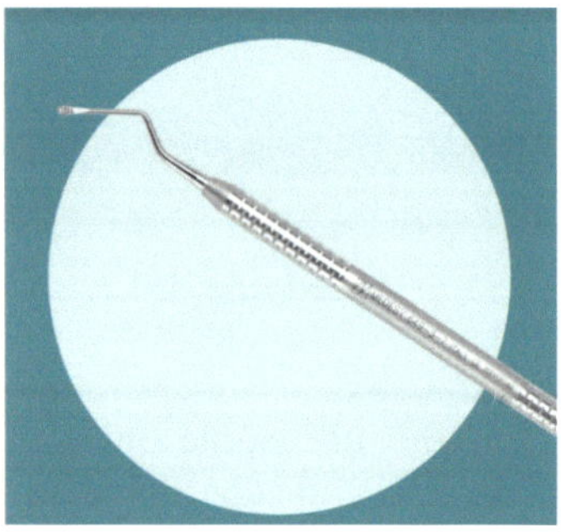

Figure 8.
Periodontal file. Hirshfield No. 3 by Hu-Friedy.

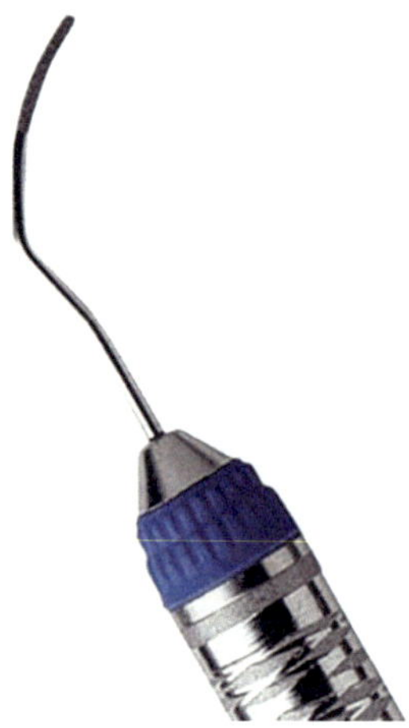

Figure 9.
Diamondtec Mesial Curette/Hu-Friedy Distal SDCM/D7.

It is worth pointing out that bacteria can reside in other areas, such as root cementum and dentin [32]. The following clinical cases illustrate the benefits of root planing supported by a careful manual technique.

In one clinical case, a 62-year-old patient presented with gingival pain, discomfort on both sides when chewing, bad breath, purulent discharge, and tooth mobility in molars 3.6 and 4.6. The patient was diagnosed with initial and moderate chronic periodontitis. In recent years, the patient had been prescribed monthly antibiotics for respiratory infections (**Figures 10–12**).

After a few weeks of non-surgical periodontal treatment, the patient improved significantly and experienced complete resolution of respiratory infections. During 10 years of periodontal maintenance, the patient did not suffer any periodontal recurrence.

The x-rays of tooth 3.6 and 4.6 show evidence of bone recovery in the furcation areas (**Figures 11** and **13**).

The second clinical case involves a 32-year-old patient, depicted in **Figures 14** and **15**, who was referred by his dentist. The patient experienced pain when chewing, spontaneous gingival bleeding, and bleeding while brushing. The diagnosis was moderate to advanced periodontitis in tooth 3.7. Periodontal treatment was performed with the Hirshfield file and the diamond tip.

After 5 months of treatment, the progress was excellent. There was no longer any tooth mobility or gingival bleeding. The evolution of the soft tissues can be seen in **Figures 16–21**.

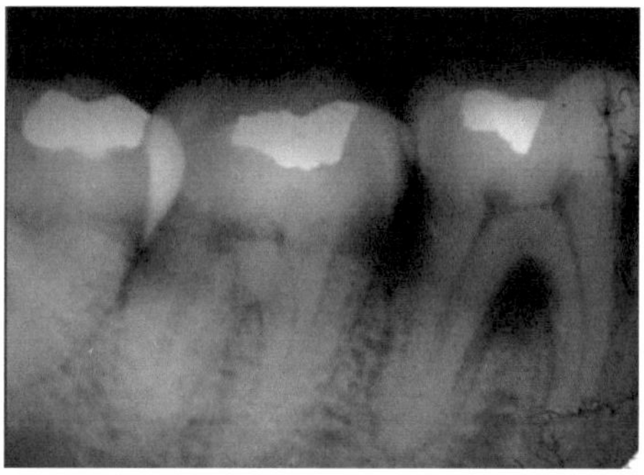

Figure 10.
X-ray of tooth 3.6 shows a radiolucent area in the furcation of the first molar.

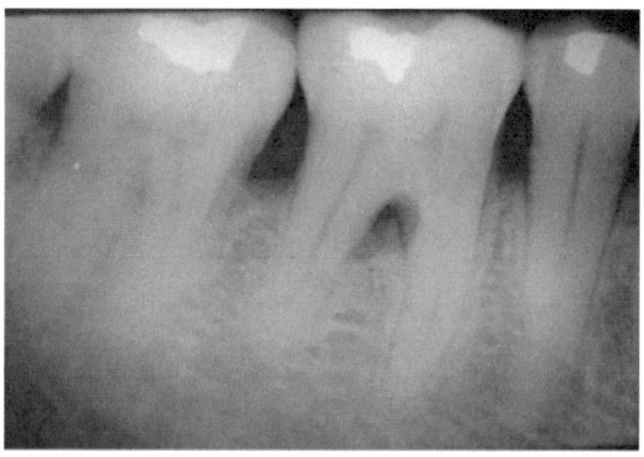

Figure 11.
Ten years after treatment the furcation area has been significantly reduced and the bone has consolidated.

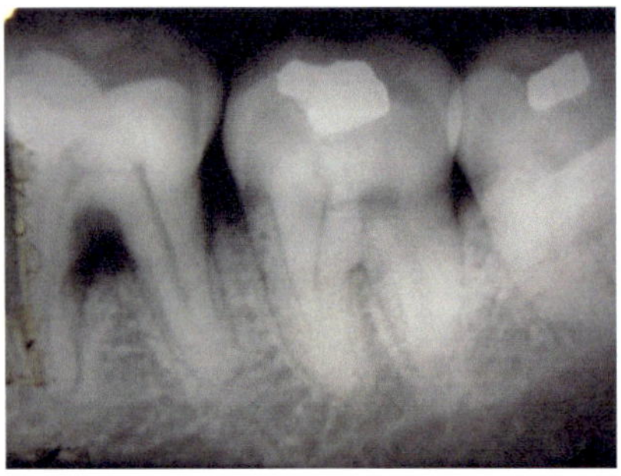

Figure 12.
The radiological image of the furcation of tooth 4.6 shows a radiolucent lesion.

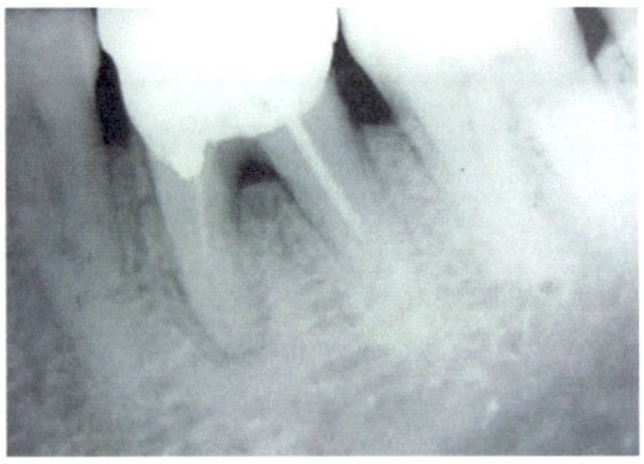

Figure 13.
Ten years after treatment the furcation lesion has reduced, and bone tissue has been regenerated.

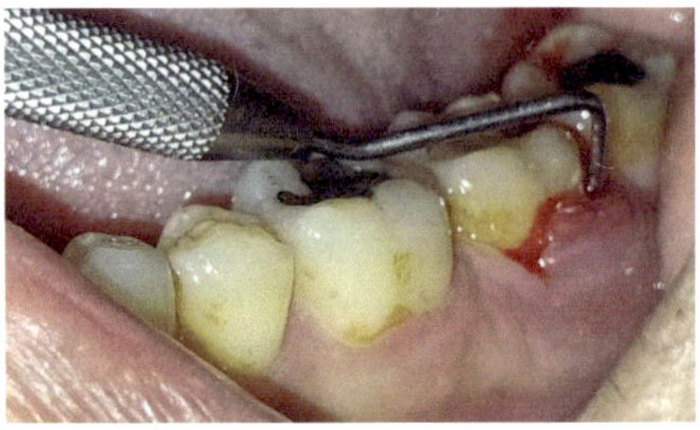

Figure 14.
In the distal area of tooth 3.7, the periodontal probe penetrates approximately 14 mm. The gingival tissues are inflamed and bleed on probing.

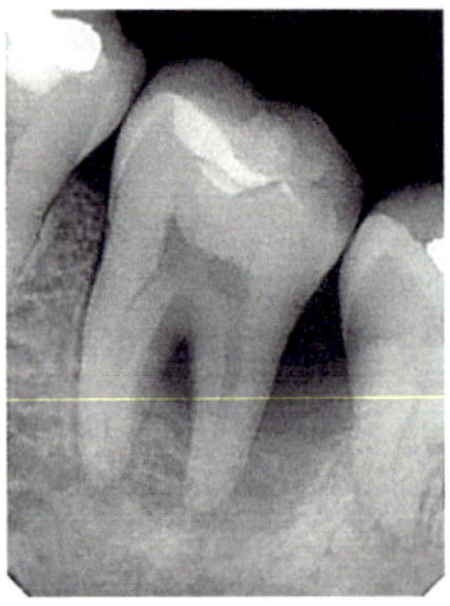

Figure 15.
The radiograph of tooth 3.7 shows bone loss up to the apex in the distal root. It also reveals bone loss in the furcation.

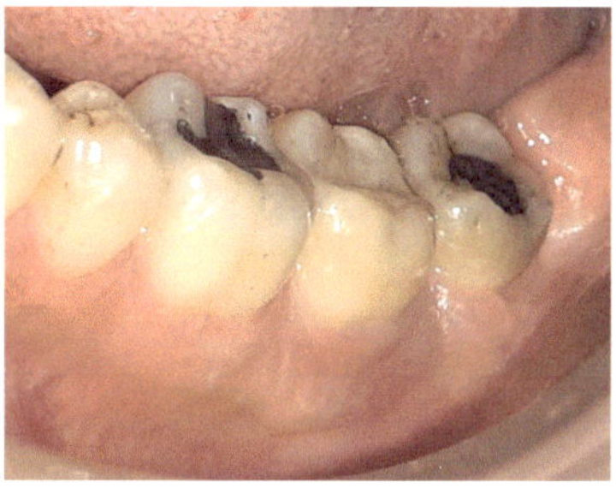

Figure 16.
The gingival tissues have recovered and show periodontal health.

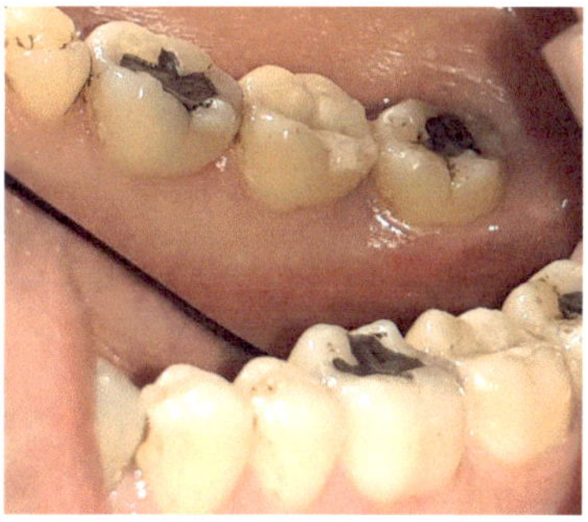

Figure 17.
The lingual side of tooth 3.7 shows periodontal health after five months of periodontal treatment.

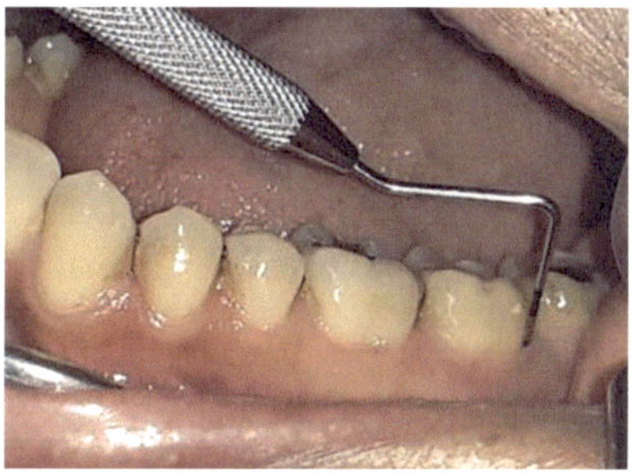

Figure 18.
In tooth 3.7, the periodontal tissues have recovered significantly. The periodontal probe enters the probing 6 mm. This probing must be very careful so as not to alter the periodontal reattachment process.

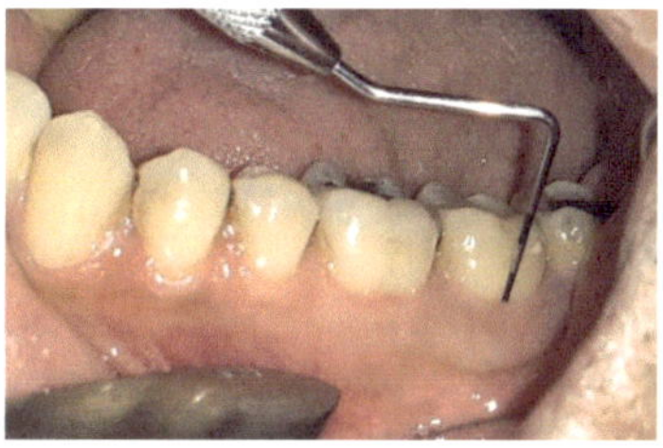

Figure 19.
In the middle part of the buccal surface near the furcation the periodontal probe enters 3 mm.

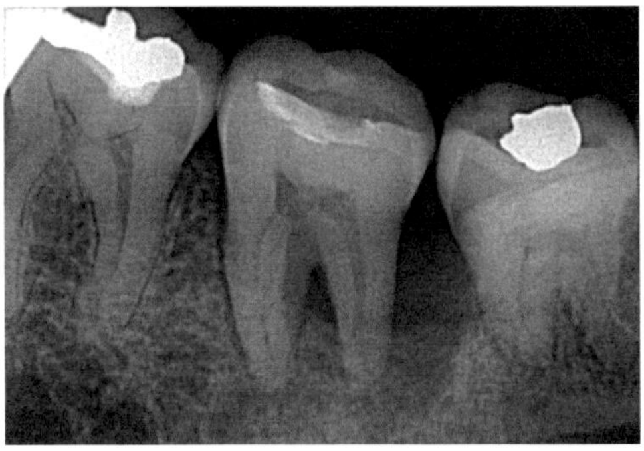

Figure 20.
The x-ray of tooth 3.7 shows recovery of the furcation and distal root. Follow-up at 5 months. The periodontal probe enters the probing 6 mm. This probing must be performed carefully to avoid altering the periodontal reattachment process.

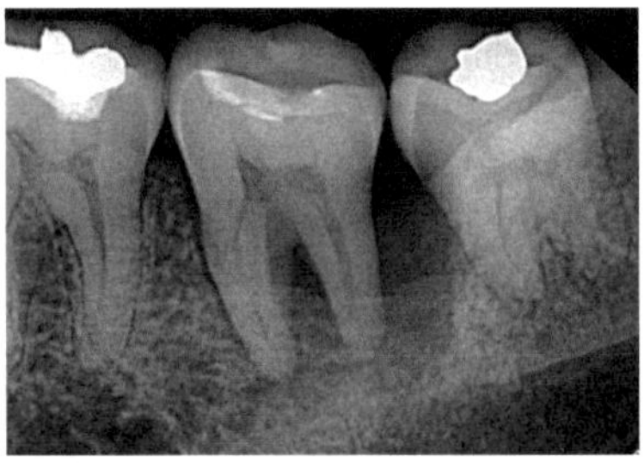

Figure 21.
Follow-up at 8 months. A consolidation of the bony structures including the furca area is observed.

5. Re-evaluation of periodontal therapy

The stone itself does not cause an inflammatory process in the periodontal pocket, but it does provide an ideal area for subgingival microbial colonization and the release and concentration of bacterial toxins. Most dental professionals have clinically experienced difficult removal of subgingival calculus, even when access is not restricted. The difficulties involved in definitively removing subgingival calculus through scaling and root planing are serious; therefore, dental appointments must be scheduled with enough time to scrupulously reevaluate the presence of subgingival calculus.

Periodontal maintenance appointments should include verification of the presence of exudate, bleeding on probing, tooth mobility, gingival color, and furcation involvement.

The bacterial communities installed inside the canals and lacunae of subgingival calculus are viable and are composed of various anaerobic gram-positive and gram-negative bacteria. Therefore, it is deduced that subgingival calculus can act as a reservoir for the continuous release of endotoxins and various microorganisms [33].

The incomplete removal of subgingival calculus creates a deposit of elements capable of producing reinfection of the periodontal pocket and recurrence of the process. This can be avoided with thorough periodontal treatment.

Another consideration to keep in mind is that cement is porous and allows the penetration and diffusion of biologically active substances from various sources, including saliva, GCF, and biofilm [16].

Scaling and root planing significantly reduces endotoxins but does not eliminate those already absorbed. In this regard, periodontal maintenance every 3 to 4 months is suggested to avoid retoxification of the treated root surfaces.

The complete removal of subgingival calculus is a challenge for any professional, including the most experienced ones. This is due to a series of factors, including restricted access, location and hardness of the subgingival calculus, irregular surfaces, bacterial penetration into the cement, and resorption gaps, among others [16].

Subgingival calculus may be strongly adhered to an area of hypermineralized cement, which would lead to incomplete removal of calculus deposits with a long formation time on the root surface [16].

A 30-year study of 375 rigorously controlled patients in a private dental clinic found a low incidence of dental caries and periodontal disease, with most patients experiencing no loss of periodontal adhesion [34].

6. Final considerations

An interesting investigation on the level of knowledge of dentists about non-surgical periodontal therapy yielded the following results:

- General practice dentists: 50% had low knowledge, 31.5% had medium knowledge, and 18.5% had high knowledge

- Dentists specialized in periodontics and implantology: 31.5 had low knowledge, 33.3% had medium knowledge, and 31.5% had high knowledge

We determined that both groups of dentists had an insufficient level of knowledge, which suggests a need to reevaluate the undergraduate curriculum in dentistry [35].

Research conducted in India examined the diagnostic knowledge, treatment strategies, and opinions of general dentists regarding periodontal treatment procedures. A questionnaire of 18 questions was administered to 100 dentists. The results showed that 64.7% of dentists responded correctly, while 85.9% believed there was a higher likelihood of recurrence in periodontal diseases and preferred extraction as a treatment option. The study concluded that dentists' knowledge is stagnant and emphasized the need to enhance the perception of periodontal treatment among general dentists in India to elevate the professional quality of their services [36].

6.1 Pointing

Manual instrumentation has the advantage of offering greater tactile sensitivity during manual scaling and root planing procedures. Similar to a systemic disease, the chronic nature of periodontal disease requires continuous monitoring and ongoing treatment [16]. The interval for patient appointments for periodontal maintenance purposes should be a function of two aspects: the severity of the disease and the patient's personal risk of recurrence [16]. Additionally, there are other periodontal treatment alternatives that can be used either as a standalone therapy or as an adjunct to non-surgical and surgical periodontal treatment. We discuss these alternatives in the sections that follow.

6.2 Ultrasonic root debridement

Ultrasonic root debridement is the removal of the calculus from root surfaces using high-frequency vibrations. Ultrasonic scraping devices produce vibrations ranging from 20,000 to 50,000 cycles per second. These instruments work by a combination of mechanical forces, irrigation, cavitation, and acoustic current forces. The ultrasonic technique allows the tip to remain in continuous rapid motion, thus preventing overheating of the tooth surface and directly contacting the calculus to remove it through elliptical, linear, or other movements, depending on the operator's technical skill and experience [37].

Ultrasonic debridement is contraindicated in patients with cardiac pacemakers. The electromagnetic field generated by the turbine can interfere with the operation of some pacemakers. Since the dentist cannot determine the type of pacemaker a patient has, ultrasonic equipment should not be used on these patients to avoid complications. Similarly, dentists and dental hygienists with pacemakers should not use ultrasonic equipment [38]. Sonic reamers, which do not generate an electromagnetic field, can be used as a substitute [39].

6.3 Air polishing systems

Air polishing is a complementary tool primarily used for removing pigmentation and supragingival plaque from teeth. It employs a compressed air system attached to a mechanized turbine that sprays an abrasive suspension against tooth surfaces. The advantages of this method include fast oral cleaning, effective removal of tartar and bacterial plaque, and painless application without unpleasant sounds. This method is particularly effective for intense pigmentation, such as that found in cigarette and pipe smokers. However, attention should be paid to drawbacks like abrasion and dust dissipation.

Due to the extensive aerosol generation by this system, it is contraindicated in patients with infectious diseases, respiratory diseases, hypertension, or those on hemodialysis [40].

6.4 Laser-assisted periodontal therapy

Lasers were introduced to dentistry in the second half of the 20th century. Their clinical applications have been expanding and there are now many FDA-approved devices for a wide variety of dental treatments [37]. Each type of laser has specific characteristics and applications depending on the wavelength and its shape [41].

In periodontics, lasers are used to eliminate calculus, reduce subgingival bacterial flora, enhance root instrumentation, and perform periodontal surgery [37].

The most common lasers for soft tissue applications are Nd:YAG, diode, erbium, and carbon dioxide lasers. These are recommended for gingival scraping over the epithelial lining of the pockets [37].

Some researchers have suggested that procedures such as incision and gum recession, gingivectomy, and biopsy can be safely performed with these lasers [42, 43]. However, there is insufficient evidence to support their use for subgingival debridement or reducing subgingival microbial values. Further research is needed to determine if scaling and root planing can be enhanced by the use of lasers [37].

Lasers are considered adjuncts to periodontal therapy when the removal of soft tissues inside the periodontal pocket is needed. Experimental studies have not shown improvement in the restoration of periodontal lesions following laser application for periodontal surgery.

While effective as an adjunct, lasers are not a substitute for conventional periodontal treatment [37]. Nonetheless, lasers represent a promising technology with a growing number of applications in dentistry [37]. Future research will help define new applications in both surgical and non-surgical therapies [37].

6.5 Photodynamic therapy

Photodynamic therapy is a non-invasive procedure that reduces morbidity and increases patient comfort. It serves as a valuable complement to scaling and root planing.

Achieving optimal periodontal health may not always be possible initially due to persistent bacterial reservoirs on the root surface. These reservoirs can be influenced by factors such as lesions in the furca, concavities, periodontal anatomical variations, mechanical limitations of instruments, and even the invasion of periodontopathogens into adjacent soft tissues or intraoral niches, necessitating repeated therapy [44].

The antibacterial effect of photodynamic therapy results from damage to the cytoplasmic membrane of bacteria, leading to membrane inactivation [45], protein and ion channel destruction, removal of critical metabolic enzymes, cell agglutination, and direct inhibition of exogenous virulence factors like lipopolysaccharides, collagenase, and proteinase [44].

Photodynamic therapy is also effective against microorganisms such as fungi, viruses, and protozoa, including the herpes simplex virus [44] and periodontopathogens like *Porphyromonas gingivalis*, *P. intermedia*, and *Aggregatibacter actinomycetemcomitans* [45, 46].

Photodynamic therapy is a good alternative to antibiotic treatments because it avoids the issue of antibiotic resistance.

6.6 Mechanical chemo debridement

Mechanical control of biofilm should be emphasized as the primary defense against periodontal disease. However, mechanical control alone is often insufficient, and thus, it is necessary to supplement with chemical agents. Using mouthwash after brushing helps control biofilm, and chlorhexidine gluconate 0.12% can reduce gingivitis and gingival bleeding. Local antimicrobials are now commonplace in non-surgical periodontal treatment.

For effective penetration into the deepest parts of periodontal pockets, antimicrobials should be administered using a syringe, soft rubber tip, or cannula.

The antimicrobial agent must meet the following requirements:

1. The drug must reach the focus of disease activity, i.e., the base of the bursa.

2. The antimicrobial should be administered in bactericidal concentration.

3. Drugs need to be kept in place on for a long time to take effect [47].

Single irrigation after scaling and root planing does not suffice for microbial suppression [48]. For example, chlorhexidine should remain in the periodontal pocket for several days to effectively interfere with biofilm repopulation.

7. Conclusion

Non-surgical periodontal treatment can stop the progression of initial and moderate periodontitis when performed with ethical standards and excellent professional practice.

Scaling and root planing procedures generally require more rigorous preparation and training during academic training.

All dentists must stay current with clinical and scientific knowledge of non-surgical periodontal therapy (scaling and root planing) due to the high prevalence of patients with periodontitis.

Minimally invasive non-surgical treatment is a promising solution and can complement existing treatment strategies for improved outcomes.

Thanks

We wish to thank Dr. Marco Moreno Asenjo from the Peruvian Association of Periodontology who passed away before this chapter was completed. He was an extraordinary friend and a great professional who promoted periodontics in Peru. We offer him our eternal gratitude.

We also thank Mg. Lily Cardich, who generously reviewed and corrected drafts of the chapter, and Miss Jennifer J. Peralta Burga, our assistant, for her excellent typing of the chapter including the changes that were made.

Conflict of interest

The authors declare that there is no conflict of interest.

Author details

Luis V. Maita Véliz*, Luis M. Maita Castañeda and María M. Castañeda Mosto
School of Dentistry, Universidad Nacional Mayor de San Marcos, Lima, Perú

*Address all correspondence to: lmaitav@unmsm.edu.pe

References

[1] Vera LV. Colegio Odontológico del Perú. Odonto antropología peruana: anomalías dentarias en cráneos de antiguos peruanos. Propaceb; 1981. Disponible en: https://books.google.com.pe/books/about/Odonto_antropolog%C3%ADa_peruana.html?id=sloeHAAACAAJ&redir_esc=y

[2] Antúnez de Mayolo S. Enfermedad periodontal en pobladores del antiguo Perú [Trabajo de investigación]. Lima: Facultad de Odontología. UNMSM. Biblioteca Nacional del Perú; 1983. Disponible en: https://www.gob.pe/institucion/bnp/buscador?contenido=todos&institucion=bnp&sheet=1&sort_by=none&term=eNFERMEDAD%20PERIODONTAL%20EN%20POBLADORES%20DEL%20ANTIGUO%20PER%C3%9A

[3] Samplonius A. Odontología antropológica: arte, ciencia e historia del alivio y curación de la patología dental en los Andes Centrales precolombinos. San Isidro, Lima, Perú: Edición del Autor; 2021. Disponible en: https://www.elvirrey.com/libro/odontologia-antropologica_70128672

[4] Caffesse RG, Mota LF, Morrison EC. The rationale for periodontal therapy. Periodontology 2000. 1995;**9**(1):7-13. DOI: 10.1111/j.1600-0757.1995.tb00051.x

[5] Cobb CM. Clinical significance of non-surgical periodontal therapy: An evidence-based perspective of scaling and root planing. Journal of Clinical Periodontology [Internet]. 2002;**29**(Suppl 2):6-16. Disponible en: https://pubmed.ncbi.nlm.nih.gov/12010523/ [Accessed: el 26 de enero de 2024]

[6] Maita Véliz L, Maita Castañeda LM. Tratamiento Periodontal no Quirúrgico, Enfoque Biológico. Odontología Sanmarquina [Internet]. 2014;**8**(1):51. Disponible en: https://revistasinvestigacion.unmsm.edu.pe/index.php/odont/article/view/3386 [Accessed: el 17 de enero de 2024]

[7] Fabrizi S, Barbieri Petrelli G, Vignoletti F, Bascones-Martínez A. Tratamiento quirúrgico vs terapia periodontal básica: estudios longitudinales en periodoncia clínica. Av Periodoncia Implantol Oral [Internet]. 2007;**19**(3):161-175. Disponible en: https://scielo.isciii.es/scielo.php?script=sci_arttext&pid=S1699-65852007000400005 [citado el 17 de enero de 2024]

[8] Maita Veliz L, Maita Castañeda LM, Castañeda MM. Chapter 1, non-surgical periodontal treatment ll: Scaling and root planning. In: Advances in Biology. Volume 4. New York: Nova Science Publishers, Inc.; 2023. Disponible en: https://novapublishers.com/?s=advances+in+biology&post_type=product

[9] Löe H, Theilade E, Jensen SB. Experimental gingivitis in man. Journal of Periodontology [Internet]. 1965;**36**(3):177-187. DOI: 10.1902/jop.1965.36.3.177

[10] Loesche WJ, Grossman NS. Periodontal disease as a specific, albeit chronic, infection: Diagnosis and treatment. Clinical Microbiology Reviews [Internet]. 2001;**14**(4):727-752. Disponible en: https://pubmed.ncbi.nlm.nih.gov/11585783/ [citado el 17 de enero de 2024]

[11] Bibi T, Khurshid Z, Rehman A, Imran E, Srivastava KC, Shrivastava D. Gingival crevicular fluid (GCF):

A diagnostic tool for the detection of periodontal health and diseases. Molecules [Internet]. 2021;**26**(5):1208. Disponible en: https://pubmed.ncbi.nlm.nih.gov/33668185/ [citado el 17 de enero de 2024]

[12] Gupta S, Chhina S, Arora SA. A systematic review of biomarkers of gingival crevicular fluid: Their predictive role in diagnosis of periodontal disease status. Journal of Oral Biology and Craniofacial Research [Internet]. 2018;**8**(2):98-104. Disponible en: https://pubmed.ncbi.nlm.nih.gov/29892530/ [citado el 17 de enero de 2024]

[13] Page RC. Peridontal disease; A new paradigm. Journal of Dental Education. 1998;**62**(10):812-821

[14] Eley BM, Cox SW. Advances in periodontal diagnosis. 5. Potential inflammatory and immune markers. British Dental Journal [Internet]. 1998;**184**(5):220-223. Disponible en: https://pubmed.ncbi.nlm.nih.gov/9581037/ [citado el 18 de enero de 2024]

[15] Cobb CM. Non-surgical pocket therapy: Mechanical. Annals of Periodontology [Internet]. 1996;**1**(1):443-490. DOI: 10.1902/annals.1996.1.1.443

[16] Cobb CM, Sottosanti JS. A re-evaluation of scaling and root planing. Journal of Periodontology [Internet]. 2021;**92**(10):1370-1378. DOI: 10.1002/jper.20-0839

[17] Marsh PD. Oral ecology, and its impact on oral microbial diversity. In: Kuramitsu KK, Ellen RP, editors. Oral Bacterial Ecology: The Molecular Basis. Norfolk: Horizon Scientific Press; 2000. pp. 11-65. Disponible en: https://www.caister.com/backlist/horizonscientificpress/ora.html

[18] Listgarten MA. The role of dental plaque in gingivitis and periodontitis. Journal of Clinical Periodontology [Internet]. 1988;**15**(8):485-487. DOI: 10.1111/j.1600-051x.1988.tb01019.x

[19] Theilade E. The experimental gingivitis studies: The microbiological perspective. Journal of Dental Research [Internet]. 1996;**75**(7):1434-1438. DOI: 10.1177/00220345960750070201

[20] Dahlén G, Lindhe J, Sato K, Hanamura H, Okamoto H. The effect of supragingival plaque control on the subgingival microbiota in subjects with periodontal disease. Journal of Clinical Periodontology [Internet]. 1992;**19**(10):802-809. DOI: 10.1111/j.1600-051x.1992.tb02174.x

[21] Hellström M-K, Ramberg P, Krok L, Lindhe J. The effect of supragingival plaque control on the subgibgival microflora in human periodontitis. Journal of Clinical Periodontology [Internet]. 1996;**23**(10):934-940. Disponible en: https://pubmed.ncbi.nlm.nih.gov/8915022/ [citado el 26 de enero de 2024]

[22] Katsanoulas T, Reneè I, Attström R. The effect of supragingival plaque control on the composition of the subgingival flora in periodontal pockets. Journal of Clinical Periodontology [Internet]. 1992;**19**(10):760-765. DOI: 10.1111/j.1600-051x.1992.tb02167.x

[23] Petersilka GJ, Ehmke B, Flemmig TF. Antimicrobial effects of mechanical debridement. Periodontology 2000 [Internet]. 2002;**28**(1):56-71. DOI: 10.1034/j.1600-0757.2002.280103.x

[24] Suvan J, Leira Y, Moreno Sancho FM, Graziani F, Derks J, Tomasi C. Subgingival instrumentation for treatment of periodontitis. A systematic review. Journal of Clinical Periodontology

[Internet]. 2020;**47**(S22):155-175. Disponible en: https://pubmed.ncbi.nlm.nih.gov/31889320/ [citado el 2 de febrero de 2024]

[25] Angst PDM, Finger Stadler A, Mendez M, Oppermann RV, van der Velden U, Gomes SC. Supportive periodontal therapy in moderate-to-severe periodontitis patients: A two-year randomized clinical trial. Journal of Clinical Periodontology [Internet]. 2019;**46**(11):1083-1093. Disponible en: https://pubmed.ncbi.nlm.nih.gov/31378975/ [citado el 2 de febrero de 2024]

[26] Maita-Véliz L, M. Maita-Castañeda L. Non-surgical treatment of periodontal diseases: Responsibilities of the dentist and the patient in periodontal therapy. En: Sridharan G, editor. Periodontology - New Insights. Londres, Inglaterra: London, UKIntechOpen; 2023.

[27] Cugini MA, Haffajee AD, Smith C, Kent RL Jr, Socransky SS. The effect of scaling and root planing on the clinical and microbiological parameters of periodontal diseases: 12-month results. Journal of Clinical Periodontology [Internet]. 2000;**27**(1):30-36. Disponible en: https://pubmed.ncbi.nlm.nih.gov/10674959/ [citado el 2 de febrero de 2024]

[28] van Winkelhof AJ, van der Velden U, de Graaff J. Microbial succession in recolonizing deep periodontal pockets after a single course of supra- and subgingival debridement. Journal of Clinical Periodontology [Internet]. 1988;**15**(2):116-122. DOI: 10.1111/j.1600-051x.1988.tb01004.x

[29] Tan BTK, Mordan NJ, Embleton J, Pratten J, Galgut PN. Study of bacterial viability within human supragingival dental calculus. Journal of Clinical Periodontology [Internet]. 2004;**75**(1):23-29. Disponible en: https://pubmed.ncbi.nlm.nih.gov/15025213/ [citado el 5 de febrero de 2024]

[30] Love RM, Jenkinson HF. Invasion of dentinal tubules by oral bacteria. Critical Reviews in Oral Biology & Medicine [Internet]. 2002;**13**(2):171-183. DOI: 10.1177/154411130201300207

[31] Giuliana G, Ammatuna P, Pizza G, Capone F, D'Angelo M. Occurrence of invading bacteria in radicular dentin of periodontally diseased teeth: Microbiological findings. Journal of Clinical Periodontology [Internet]. 1997;**24**(7):478-485. DOI: 10.1111/j.1600-051x.1997.tb00215.x

[32] Adriaens PA, De Boever JA, Loesche WJ. Bacterial invasion in root cementum and radicular dentin of periodontally diseased teeth in humans: A reservoir of periodontopathic bacteria. Journal of Periodontology [Internet]. 1988;**59**(4):222-230. Disponible en: https://pubmed.ncbi.nlm.nih.gov/3164373/ [citado el 5 de febrero de 2024]

[33] McCoy SA, Creamer HR, Kawanami M, Adams DF. The concentration of lipopolysaccharide on individual root surfaces at varying times following in vivo root planing. Journal of Periodontology [Internet]. 1987;**58**(6):393-399. Disponible en: https://pubmed.ncbi.nlm.nih.gov/3298609/ [citado el 9 de febrero de 2024]

[34] Axelsson P, Nyström B, Lindhe J. The long-term effect of a plaque control program on tooth mortality, caries and periodontal disease in adults: Results after 30 years of maintenance. Journal of Clinical Periodontology [Internet]. 2004;**31**(9):749-757. Disponible en: https://pubmed.ncbi.nlm.nih.gov/15312097/ [citado el 14 de febrero de 2024]

[35] Bocanegra R. Nivel de conocimiento de los odontólogos acerca de la terapia periodontal no quirúrgica. Tesis estomatológica de especialidad Periodoncia e Implantología. Peru: Universidad Peruana Cayetano Heredia; 2019. Disponible en: https://repositorio.upch.edu.pe/bitstream/handle/20.500.12866/5952/Nivel_BocanegraArista_Rocio.pdf?sequence=1&isAllowed=y

[36] Sathyamurthy P, Padhye A, Gupta H. Knowledge of diagnosis, treatment strategies, and opinions on periodontal treatment procedures among general dentists in an Indian urban population: A questionnaire survey. Journal of Indian Association of Public Health Dentistry [Internet]. 2018;**16**(1):62. Disponible en: https://www.jiaphd.org/temp/JIndianAssocPublicHealthDent16162-7784895_213728.pdf

[37] Beemsterboer PL, Perry DA, Essex G. Periodontología para el higienista dental. 4ta edición ed. Barcelona, España: Elsevier Inc.; 2014. Disponible en: https://app.bibguru.com/p/b193b403-ddc3-458a-8d0a-3653003cf561

[38] Adams D, Fulford N, Beechy J, MacCarthy J, Stephens M. The cardiac pacemaker and ultrasonic scalers. British Dental Journal [Internet]. 1982;**152**(5):171-173. Disponible en: https://pubmed.ncbi.nlm.nih.gov/7041930/ [citado el 23 de abril de 2024]

[39] Drisko CL, Cochran DL, Blieden T, Bouwsma OJ, Cohen RE, Damoulis P, et al. Sonic and ultrasonic scalers in periodontics*. Journal of Periodontology [Internet]. 2000;**71**(11):1792-1801. Disponible en: https://pubmed.ncbi.nlm.nih.gov/11128930/ [citado el 23 de abril de 2024]

[40] Barnes CM. Extrinsic stain removal. In: Clinical Practice of the Dental Hygienist. 11th ed. Editorial: Wolters Kluwer Health Adis (ESP) 2013. pp. 689-708. Disponible en: https://experts.nebraska.edu/en/publications/extrinsic-stain-removal

[41] Dederich DN, Bushick RD. Lasers in dentistry. Journal of the American Dental Association [Internet]. 2004;**135**(2):204-212. Disponible en: https://pubmed.ncbi.nlm.nih.gov/15005437/ [citado el 26 de abril de 2024]

[42] Frentzen M, Braun A, Aniol D. Er:YAG laser scaling of diseased root surfaces. Journal of Periodontology [Internet]. 2002;**73**(5):524-530. Disponible en: https://pubmed.ncbi.nlm.nih.gov/12027255/ [citado el 26 de abril de 2024]

[43] Schwarz F, Sculean A, Rothamel D, Schwenzer K, Georg T, Becker J. Clinical evaluation of an Er:YAG laser for nonsurgical treatment of peri-implantitis: A pilot study. Clinical Oral Implants Research [Internet]. 2005;**16**(1):44-52. Disponible en: https://pubmed.ncbi.nlm.nih.gov/15642030/ [citado el 26 de abril de 2024]

[44] Gómez Hernández C, Domínguez Martín A, García Kass AI, García Núñez JA. Aplicación complementaria de terapia fotodinámica y de la radiación láser de Er:YAG al tratamiento no quirúrgico de la periodontitis crónica: estudio comparativo de sus efectos clínicos, antiinflamatorios y antimicrobianos. Av Odontoestomatol [Internet]. 2011;**27**(3):147-160. Disponible en: https://scielo.isciii.es/scielo.php?script=sci_arttext&pid=S0213-12852011000300005 [citado el 26 de abril de 2024]

[45] Haas R, Dörtbudak O, Mensdorff-pouilly N, Mailath G. Elimination of bacteria on different implant surfaces through photosensitization and soft laser.

An in vitro study. Clinical Oral Implants Research [Internet]. 1997;**8**(4):249-254. Disponible en: https://pubmed.ncbi.nlm.nih.gov/9586470/ [citado el 26 de abril de 2024]

[46] de Oliveira RR, Schwartz-Filho HO, Novaes AB Jr, Taba M Jr. Antimicrobial photodynamic therapy in the non-surgical treatment of aggressive periodontitis: A preliminary randomized controlled clinical study. Journal of Periodontology [Internet]. 2007;**78**(6):965-973. Disponible en: https://pubmed.ncbi.nlm.nih.gov/17539707/ [citado el 26 de abril de 2024]

[47] Greenstein G. Subgingival irrigation--an adjunct to periodontal therapy. Current status and future directions. Journal of Dental Hygiene [Internet]. 1990;**64**(8):389-397. Disponible en: https://pubmed.ncbi.nlm.nih.gov/2090788/ [citado el 26 de abril de 2024]

[48] Bonito AJ, Lux L, Lohr KN. Impact of local adjuncts to scaling and root planing in periodontal disease therapy: A systematic review. Journal of Periodontology [Internet]. 2005;**76**(8):1227-1236. Disponible en: https://pubmed.ncbi.nlm.nih.gov/16101353/ [citado el 26 de abril de 2024]